Environmental Health - Management and Prevention Practices

Edited by Abdelhadi Makan

Published in London, United Kingdom

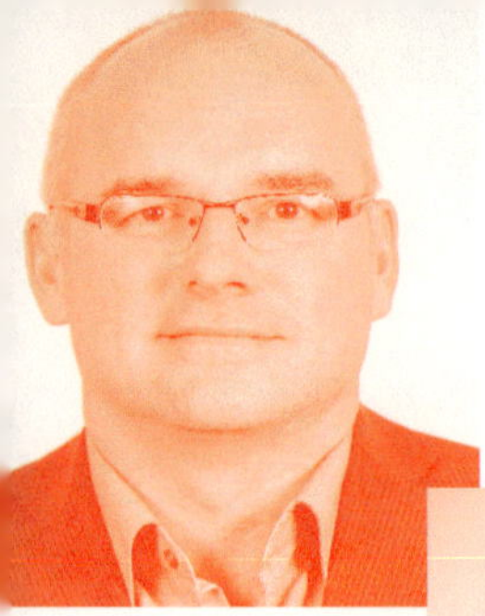
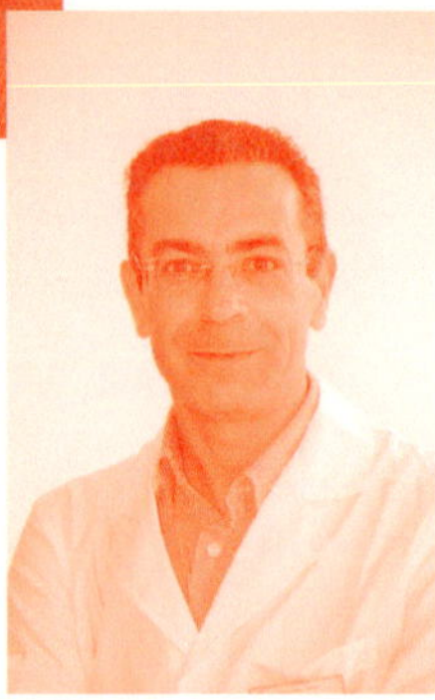
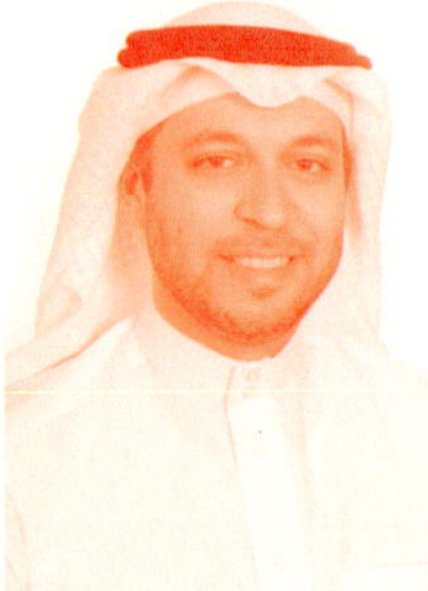
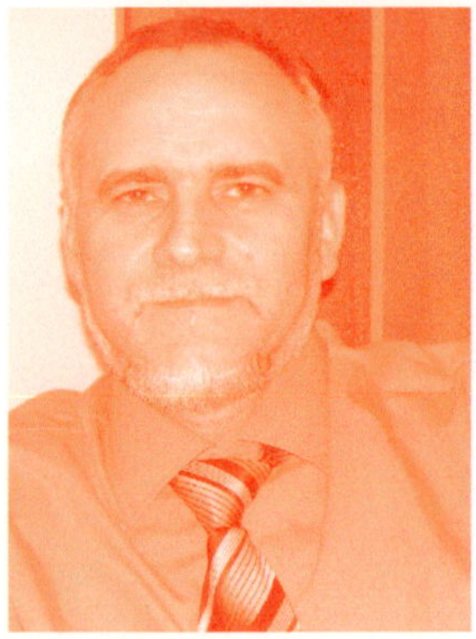
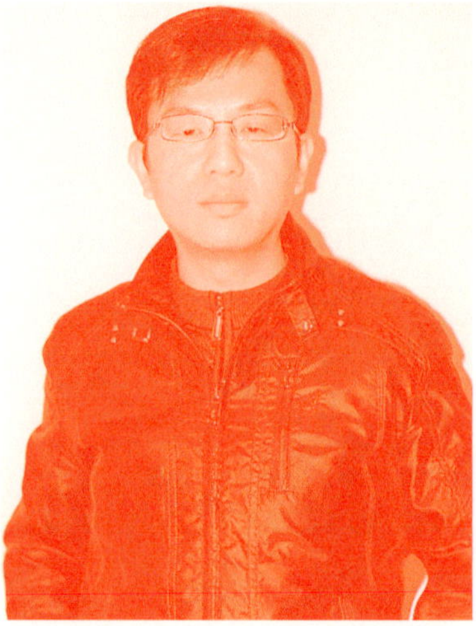
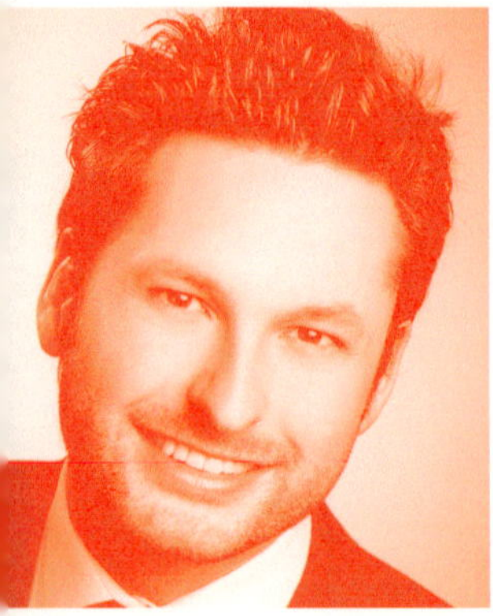
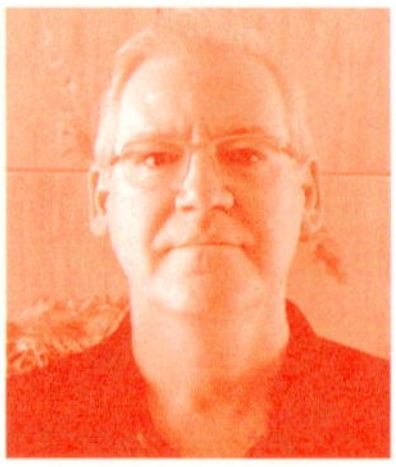

IntechOpen

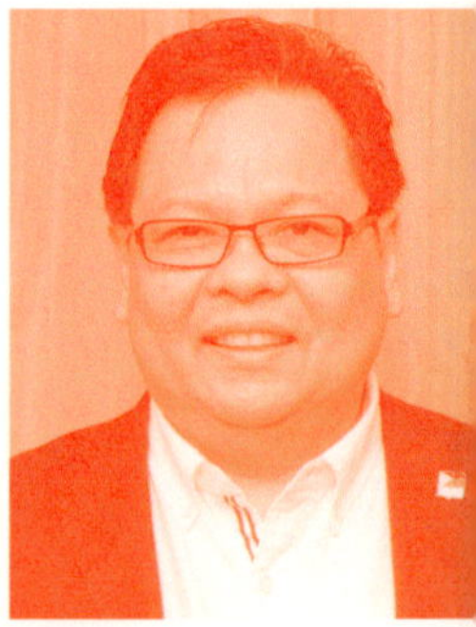
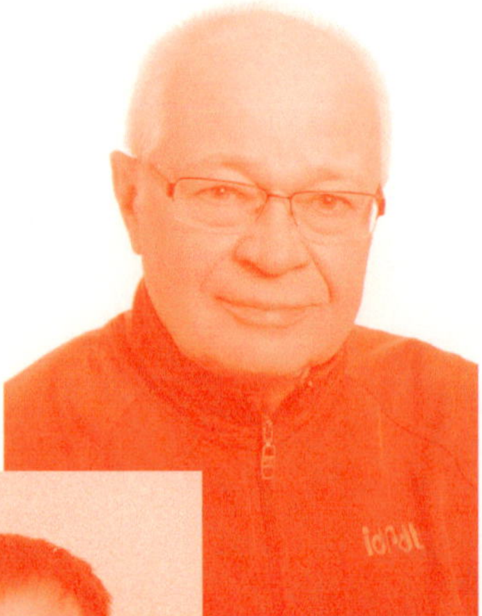
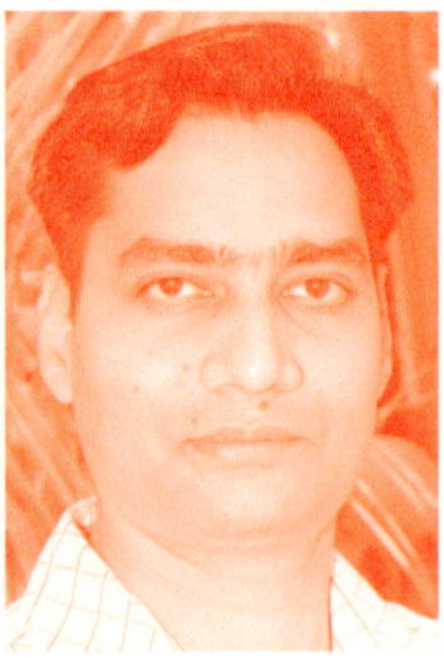
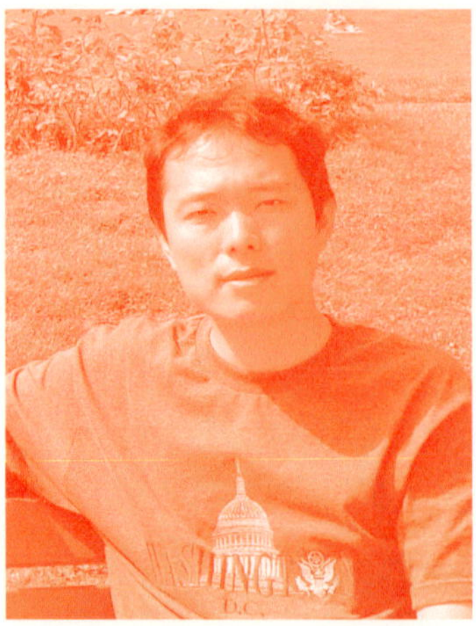
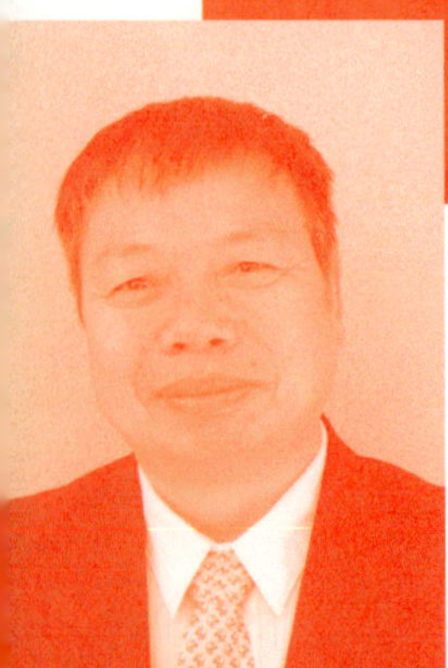
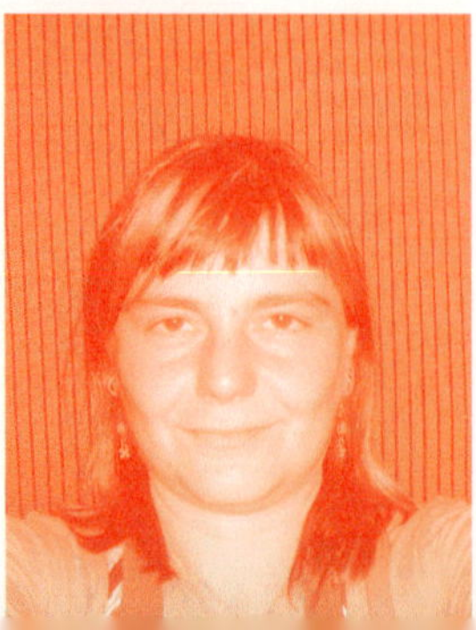

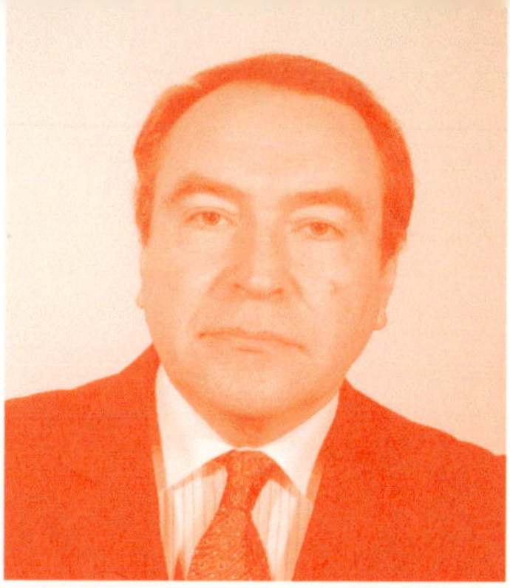
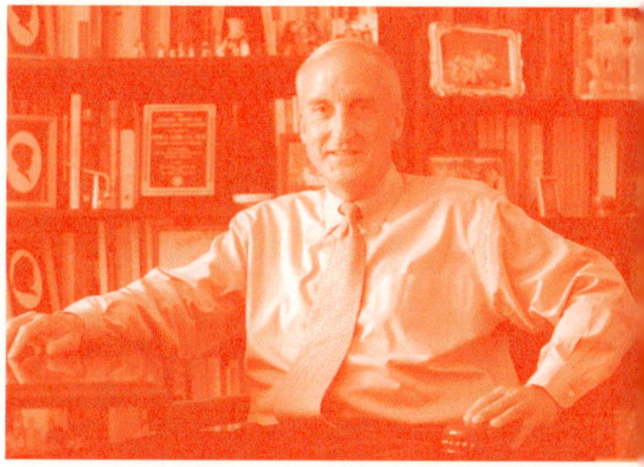
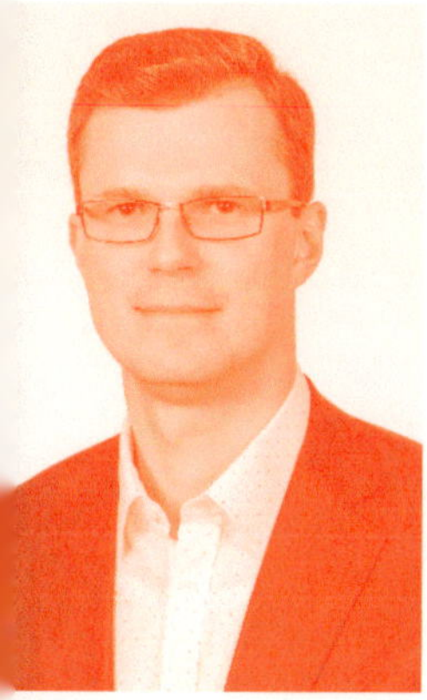
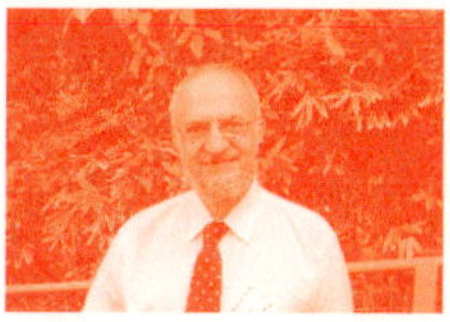
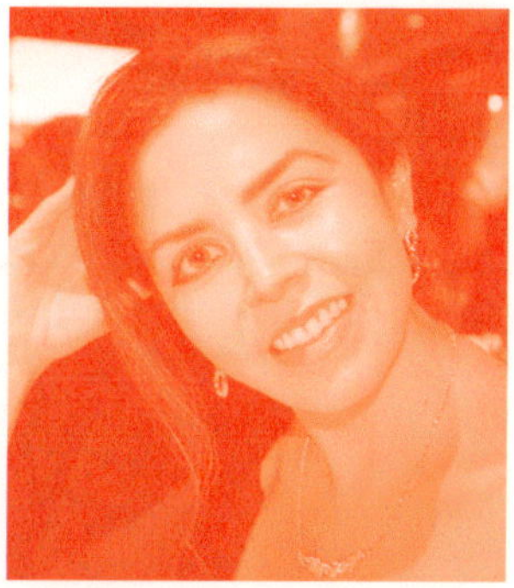

Supporting open minds since 2005

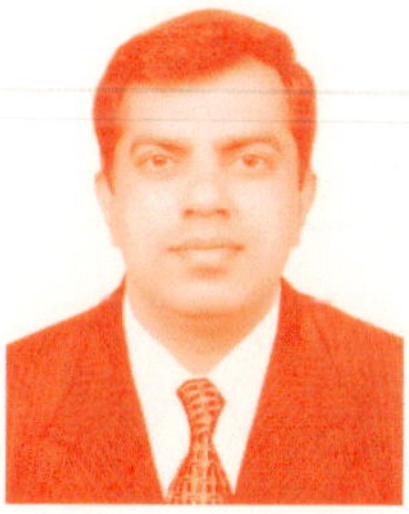
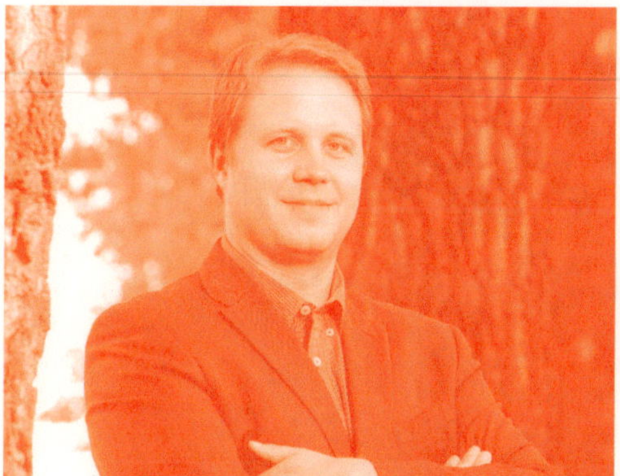
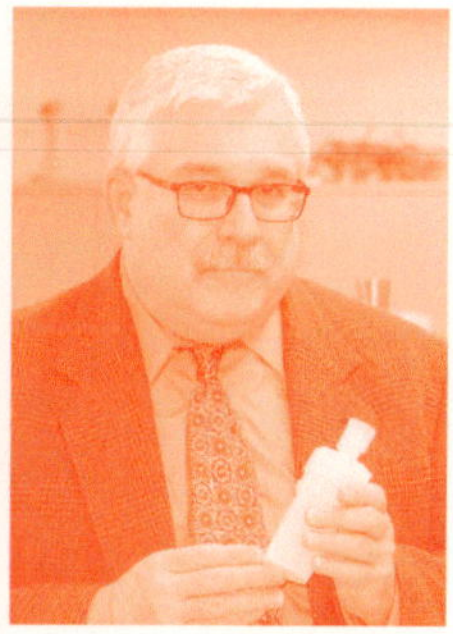
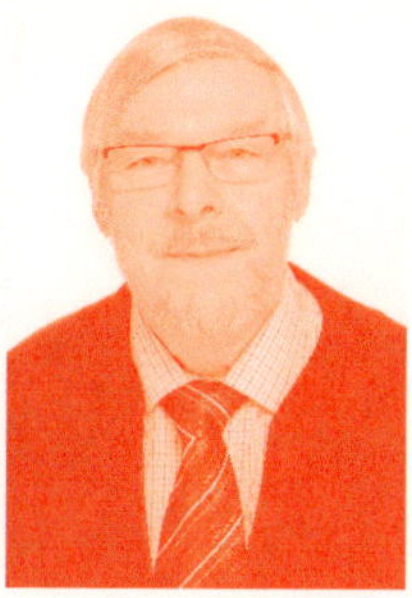
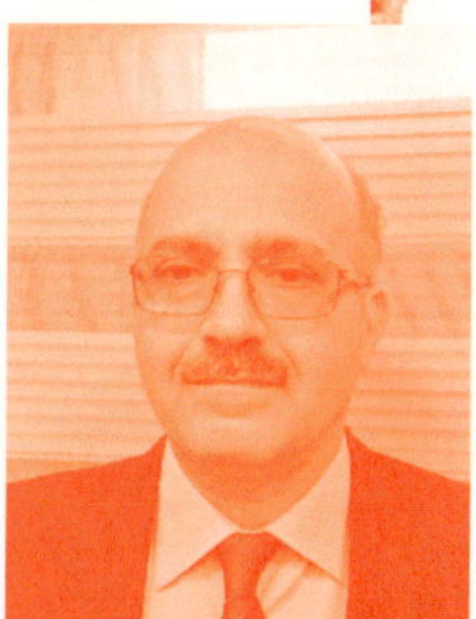
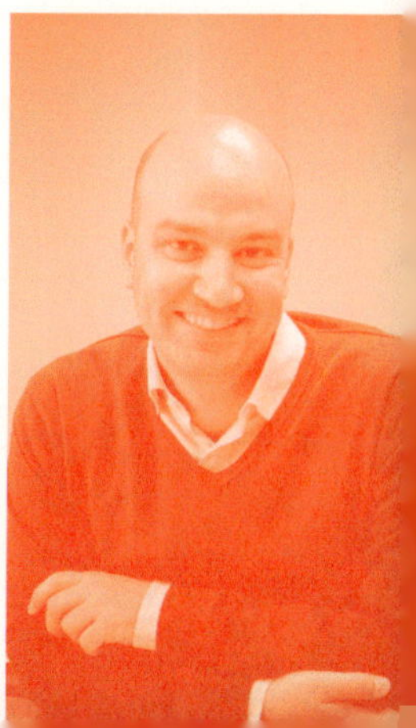
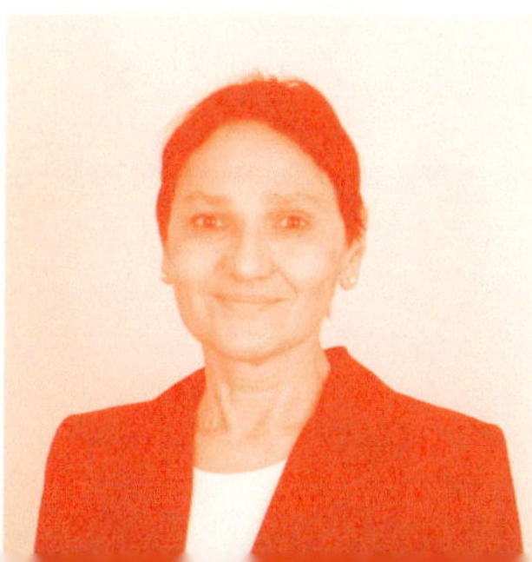

Environmental Health - Management and Prevention Practices
http://dx.doi.org/10.5772/intechopen.73403
Edited by Abdelhadi Makan

Contributors
Calvin Atewamba, Edward R Rhodes, Mirzi Betasolo, Dominika Saniewska, Kurt Buchmann, Lyda Espitia - Pérez, Luisa Jimenez - Vidal, Pedro Juan Espitia - Pérez, Diana Linhares, Patricia Garcia, Armindo Rodrigues, Ketty Balthazard-Accou, Evens Emmanuel, Patrice Agnamey, Christian Raccurt

First published in London, United Kingdom, 2020 by IntechOpen
IntechOpen is the global imprint of INTECHOPEN LIMITED, registered in England and Wales, registration number: 11086078, 7th floor, 10 Lower Thames Street, London, EC3R 6AF, United Kingdom
Printed in Croatia

British Library Cataloguing-in-Publication Data
A catalogue record for this book is available from the British Library

Additional hard and PDF copies can be obtained from orders@intechopen.com

Environmental Health - Management and Prevention Practices
Edited by Abdelhadi Makan
p. cm.
Print ISBN 978-1-78984-894-6
Online ISBN 978-1-78984-895-3
eBook (PDF) ISBN 978-1-83962-777-4

For EU product safety concerns:
IN TECH d.o.o., Prolaz Marije Krucifikse Kozulić 3, 51000 Rijeka, Croatia, info@intechopen.com or visit our website at intechopen.com.

Meet the editor

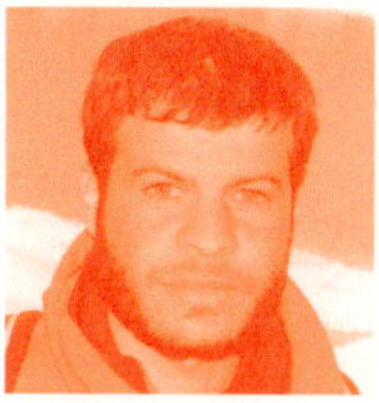

Abdelhadi Makan has a PhD in Waste Management and Environmental Sciences. He gained relevant professional experience in fields such as environmental science, chemistry, and waste management. Through all his academic and professional publications, he has fully practiced both qualitative and quantitative research methods. Additionally, he is the founder and CEO of ENQUAS Consulting, which is an investigation and consultancy office practicing in environmental, quality, and safety domains. Currently, he works as a full-time professor at the National School of Applied Sciences (ENSAH), Abdelmalek Essaâdi University, Morocco. In his spare time, he acts as editorial board member, reviewer, and proofreader for several reputed scientific journals.

Contents

Preface

It took a long time for humans to recognize the existence of a direct link between environmental pollution and health deterioration. In the 1990s, scientists demonstrated the existence of this link through epidemiological studies and new technical materials, which can measure accumulation effects of small toxic quantities. As a result, concerns about human health were accentuated, and the notion of environmental health has emerged. In fact, the environment does not act in the same way on each individual. A healthy person can adapt more easily to external constraints. However, for a sick, malnourished, or stressed person, the capacity to adapt is reduced and health will degrade more quickly.

Generally, this book deals with aspects of human health, such as quality of life, which are determined by physical, chemical, biological, and social factors of the environment. It covers a few policies and practices for managing, controlling, and preventing environmental factors that may affect the health of current and future generations. Specifically, the book is organized into seven main topics related either to the natural environment or to the built environment. These include, namely, air and water pollution, rainwater harvesting, climate change effects, marine pollution, and ecological indicators.

- **Chapter 1** reviews the main characteristics of particulate matters (PM), their effects on health, and their role in genomic instability. Additionally, it explores different biomarkers associated with PM exposure, DNA damage, and the influence of PM-related oxidative stress in disease development.

- **Chapter 2** examines the biological cycle and physicochemical behavior of Cryptosporidium oocysts in order to understand their movement through soils, and to evaluate the chemical conditions and soil characteristics, which can constitute factors influencing the retention of oocysts or facilitate their transfer into groundwater.

- **Chapter 3** investigates rainwater harvesting infrastructure management, which is a promising alternative in the imminence of increasing water scarcity and escalating demand for water supply. It maximizes water efficiency and minimizes the environmental impact. Additionally, a rainwater harvesting system may increase water availability, self-reliance, and sustainability.

- **Chapter 4** covers the main effects of fluoride exposure on the human body and discusses the use of a multidisciplinary approach that brings together the geoscience, biomedical, and public health communities to address environmental health problems.

- **Chapter 5** assesses biophysical and economic factors of climate change impacts on the agriculture sector of the Economic Community of West African States, mainly during the decade that follows the launching of the Comprehensive Africa Agricultural Development Programme and Maputo Accord.

- **Chapter 6** constructs a multi-year mass balance of mercury in the Gulf of Gdańsk. This mass balance can be used to identify and better understand the dominant mercury sources and sinks in the gulf and can provide an initial basis for future research in the region.

- Finally, **Chapter 7** explores Baltic parasites and recommends the ones that can be used as biological indicators. The recommended indicator parasites comprise trematodes (*Cryptocotyle lingua*, *Diplostomum spathaceum*, *Lepidapedon elongatum*, *Hemiurus lühei*, *Brachyphallus crenatus*), nematodes (*Hysterothylacium aduncum*, *Contracaecum osculatum*, *Anisakis simplex*, *Pseudoterranova decipiens*, *Capillaria gracilis*), and acanthocephalans (*Echinorhynchus gadi*, *Corynosoma spp.*, *Pomphorhynchus laevis*).

Abdelhadi Makan
Professor,
National School of Applied Sciences – Al Hoceima,
Abdelmalek Essaâdi University,
Morocco

Chapter 1

Particulate Matter Exposure: Genomic Instability, Disease, and Cancer Risk

Lyda Espitia-Pérez, Luisa Jiménez-Vidal and Pedro Espitia-Pérez

Abstract

The United Nations Environment Programme (UNEP/WHO) defines particulate matter (PM) as a mixture of solid or liquid particles suspended and dispersed in the air. Constituted by a complex mixture of organic and inorganic components like metals, acids, soil, and dust is considered a major human carcinogen present in air pollution. When inhaled, PM particles penetrate the respiratory tract, where they affect different organs and systems depending on their aerodynamic size and chemical properties. In the organism, this cocktail-like mixture can interact with cellular mechanisms related to the production of reactive oxygen species (ROS) and can cause damage to important macromolecules such as DNA, lipids, and proteins. Additionally, PM induces a variety of effects at a cellular level, such as inflammation, DNA damage, and genomic instability, acting as a driving force of carcinogenic processes and increasing the incidence of respiratory, cardiopulmonary, neurogenerative, and neurodevelopment disorders. This book chapter reviews the main characteristics of PM, its effects on health, and its role in genomic instability and associated molecular mechanisms. Additionally, we explore different biomarkers associated with PM exposure, DNA damage, and the influence of PM-related oxidative stress in disease development.

Keywords: $PM_{1.0}$, $PM_{2.5}$, PM_{10}, cancer, genomic instability

1. Introduction

Air pollution represents a worldwide problem with a significant impact on ecosystems and human health. According to the World Health Organization (WHO), air pollution poses the main environmental risk to health [1]. According to the International Agency for Research on Cancer (IARC), exposure to particulate matter (PM) in air pollution is considered as a human carcinogen [2]. PM is constituted by a heterogeneous mixture of a large variety of small particles of solids and liquids of both organic and inorganic nature, derived from natural and anthropogenic sources. PM size is an important factor that influences how it is deposited in the respiratory tract and affects human health. Large particles are generally filtered in the nose and throat and do not necessarily cause problems. An important fraction of PM is referred to as PM_{10}, composed of particles ≤ 10 μm. PM_{10} is generally subdivided into a fraction of finer particles ≤ 2.5 μm ($PM_{2.5}$) and a coarser fraction of particles >2.5

and <10 μm ($PM_{2.5–10}$). $PM_{2.5}$ is dominated by products of combustion and secondary particles, while $PM_{2.5–10}$ consists mainly of crustal, biological, and fine particle fraction components [3]. Thus, smaller PM particles can penetrate deeply in the lungs, activating molecular mechanisms of epithelial and defense cells [4].

Exposure to PM, especially around industrial zones and mining systems, has been associated with an increase in the morbidity of respiratory diseases, certain types of allergies, cardiopulmonary diseases, neurological disorders, and some types of cancer [5]. The biological mechanisms behind these associations are not entirely known, but the results of toxicological studies in vitro and in vivo have shown that PM induces several adverse cellular effects due to the synergistic generation of reactive oxygen species (ROS), which includes genotoxicity, mutagenicity, oxidative stress, inflammation, and increased DNA damage potentially associated with genomic instability [6].

Genomic instability is defined as a cell's increased likelihood to develop and accumulate genome alterations (mutations, chromosomal alterations, epigenetic/posttranscriptional modifications, and changes in gene expression). The frequency of these alterations is related to the loss of fidelity in mechanisms such as DNA replication, chromosomal segregation, DNA repair, and cell cycle progression [7]. These alterations are capable of acting as a driving force of the carcinogenic process, a reason why PM exposures are associated with an increase in cancer risk [6]. This cancer risk can be evaluated through measurable changes (biochemical, physiological, or morphological) that associate with toxic exposure or any early biochemical alteration. The identification of these genome damage biomarkers is useful by defining a pathogenesis state, such as cancer. It is also of vital importance for disease prevention [8]. Consequently, the toxicological investigation of complex mixtures such as PM is one of the main objectives of recent research in toxicology and cancer [9]. In order to elucidate how genomic background and PM exposure can interact, this book chapter focuses on reviewing relevant information based on the three main aspects: *(I) the characteristics of PM as an environmental pollutant and its effects on health*, *(II) the molecular mechanisms of the cellular effects associated with genomic instability by PM exposure*, and *(III) the use of different risk biomarkers based on the determination of chromosomal instability for estimation of cancer risk in populations exposed to PM.*

2. Environmental air pollution, PM, and health effects

Environmental air pollution is defined as the presence in the atmosphere of contaminating elements that alter its composition and that affect any component of the ecosystem [10]. Air pollution is constituted by an extremely complex mixture that includes inorganic components (sulfates, nitrates, ammonium, chloride, and trace metals), elemental and organic carbon, biological components (bacteria, spores, and pollens), and adsorbed volatile and semi-volatile organic compounds. Besides, environmental particles, when mixed with atmospheric gases (ozone, sulfur nitric oxides, and carbon monoxide) can generate environmental aerosols or PM [11].

PM is a complex mixture of solid and liquid particles of different origin, size, shape, and chemical composition [12]. Atmospheric PM comes from a variety of emission sources, including natural and anthropogenic sources. In addition, the particulate material can be emitted directly into the atmosphere (primary particles) or formed in the atmosphere from gaseous precursors (secondary particles) [13]. Among the emission sources, industries are considered one of the most significant anthropogenic sources of trace metals [14, 15] although traffic emissions could also be regarded as an important source of PM and metals in urban atmospheres [16, 17].

The size of the PM is of great interest to understand their mobility and their impact on health. The respiratory system is the primary intake route of PM in the body, and the deposition of particles in different parts of the human body depends on the size, shape, and density of the particles, as well as on the individual's breathing (nasal or oral) [10]. Such health effects induced in the organism depend on the granulometry, morphology, time of exposure, individual susceptibility, and finally the chemical composition of the particles [18]. In terms of size, PM is categorized according to aerodynamic size and is divided into three main groups: the first group is large particles, which are generally filtered in the nose and throat and do not necessarily cause problems. The second group is PM_{10}, an essential fraction of PM mostly produced by mechanical processes and with sizes between 2.5 and 10 micrometers (μm). PM_{10} is also called "coarse fraction" or "breathable fraction" because of its ability to enter the respiratory tract [19]. Finally, the third group is $PM_{2.5}$ or "fine fraction" whose aerodynamic diameter is ≤2.5 μm. $PM_{2.5}$ is mainly derived from combustion sources, such as automobiles, trucks, and other vehicle exhausts, as well as from stationary combustion sources [19]. $PM_{2.5}$ can easily reach the terminal bronchioles and alveoli, from where can be phagocytosed by alveolar macrophages and cross the capillary-alveolar barrier to be transported to other organs by blood circulation [20].

Recently, "ultrafine" particles have been described with aerodynamic size <0.1 μm; these particles are generated by photochemical processes and combustion, also from various natural and anthropogenic sources, and can go directly from the alveoli to the bloodstream [21]. Besides, their smaller size and higher surface/mass ratio may allow them to have more bioavailability for bioreactive chemicals in their large surface, allowing greater access to the contact points of the cells, increasing its toxicity.

Chemically, PM mainly comprises ions, reactive gases, salts (sulfates, nitrates), organic compounds such as polycyclic and/or inorganic aromatic hydrocarbons (PAHs), heavy metals (i.e., Fe, Cu, Mo, V, and those with high toxicity such as Pb, Cd, and Ni), and carbon core particle [22] compounds with known genotoxic, mutagenic, and/or carcinogenic activity. However, the chemical composition of PM varies greatly and depends on numerous geographical, meteorological, and source-specific variables [11]. PM can absorb and transfer a myriad of pollutants which results in its variable composition, so depending on the source and composition of the PM, different subsets of components may be found on different fractions. PM_{10} and $PM_{2.5}$ are dominated by mechanically abraded or grinded particles including finely divided minerals such as oxides of aluminum silicate, iron, calcium, and potassium [23]. $PM_{2.5}$ comprises the soot-rich fraction and other particles within the atmospheric gas phase resulting in subsequent agglomeration of PM and producing inorganic ions such as sulfate, nitrate, and ammonia, as well as carbon combustion residues, organic aerosols, metals, and other combustion products. Unlike inorganic elements that can be present in both $PM_{2.5}$ and PM_{10} fractions, PAHs show a strong association with the $PM_{2.5}$ fraction. Several studies have reported that 87–95% of PAHs can be found in the $PM_{2.5}$ fraction [24]. The latter correlation seems to be stronger for the heavier and more carcinogenic PAHs with five and six aromatic rings.

Also, coarse and fine fractions differ with ultrafine particles in composition regarding various heavy metals and possibly a higher content of compounds with redox activity, such as prooxidant PAHs (dibenzo (a,l) pyrene) [25] (**Table 1**).

Health effects caused by PM exposure are supported by increasingly a growing number of scientific evidences. The latter comes from a variety of epidemiological studies using both population and occupational approach for assessing PM exposure, alongside with toxicological studies and human-controlled exposure experiments. Results support the causal relationship between PM and premature death, increased morbidity from respiratory diseases [26], lung cancer [27], and cardiopulmonary diseases [28]. In fact, several health-related studies indicate a strong association of

Study area	Population description	Area description	Analyzed pollutants	Reference
Aracaju, Brazil	Urban	Metropolitan	PM, SO_2, and elements (Cu, Fe, Mn, Ni, V, and Ti)	[33]
Beijing, China	Urban	Metropolitan	PM (PM2.5), NOx, SO_2, volatile organic compounds (HAPs), ozone, nitrate	[34, 35]
Guajira, Colombia	Ethnical	Semi-arid	PM (PM10 and PM2.5), extractable organic matter (apolar and polar fractions), and elements (Al, Cl, Cr, Cu, K, Mg, Mn, Na, P, S, Si, Ti, and Zn)	[36]
Houston, USA	Urban	Metropolitan	PM2.5, NOx, volatile organic compounds (light alkenes), ozone, sulfate	[37, 38]
Huelva, Spain	Urban	Industrial	PM (PM10, PM2.5 and PM1), phosphate, and As	[2]
Los Angeles, USA	Urban	Metropolitan	PM (PM2.5), NOx, volatile organic compounds (HAPs), ozone, nitrate	[39, 40]
	Urban	Metropolitan	PM2.5, organic carbon, ammonium, nitrate, sulfate, and elements (Al, Br, Ca, Cl, Cu, Fe, K, Mn, Na, Ni, Pb, Si, V, Zn)	[41, 42]
Mexico City, Mexico	Urban	Metropolitan	PM (PM2.5), NOx, volatile organic compounds (alkanes, HAPs), ozone, sulfate	[43–45]
Sao Paulo and Piracicaiba, Brazil	Urban	Metropolitan	PM (PM10 and PM2.5), sulphate, nitrate, ammonium, elemental carbon, and particulate organic material	[46]

Table 1.
Particulate matter characterization from several cohort studies worldwide.

airborne PM generated around coal mines with adverse impacts such as increased cardiovascular disease and other pathologies such as pneumoconiosis, neurodegenerative and neurodevelopment disorders, and different types of cancer [21].

Particularly, it has been described that PM_{10} exposure can cause deterioration of the respiratory function in a short term, whereas in the long term, it is associated with the development of chronic diseases, cancer, or premature death. On the other hand, $PM_{2.5}$ exhibits a strong association with increased risk of respiratory disease, cardiovascular disorders, type II diabetes mellitus, and even autism spectrum disorders [29–31]. Finally, ultrafine particles may be the most active in terms of the induction of systemic effects; in fact, studies describe the role of ultrafine particles in the increased risk of cardiac hospitalization due to early myocardial infarction and increased frequency of readmissions for patients who have survived myocardial infarction and heart failure, which allows to consider $PM_{2.5}$ as a risk factor for cardiovascular disease [32].

3. Genomic instability by PM exposure and its relation with carcinogenesis

Several studies have examined in different experimental models in vivo and in vitro the effects of exposure to coarse, fine, and ultrafine PM. These studies provide biological support to epidemiological studies that show an association between acute exposure to PM and health effects. The relationship between disease and air pollution is well established, but the molecular mechanism regarding their relationship is yet to be fully explored.

The interaction of PM with the cellular plasma membrane and its receptors and ion channels may directly trigger a biological response. The most important pathophysiological mechanism that has been proposed to explain the association of PM exposure and occurrence of respiratory infections, cancer, and chronic cardiopulmonary diseases is oxidative stress through the generation of ROS. ROS are oxygen-related compounds able to induce changes in cellular redox cycle and therefore triggering a series of events in cascade such as inflammation, apoptosis, and oxidative damage to macromolecules such as proteins, lipids, and nucleic acids [33]. Under the name of ROS, several species derived from the reduction of molecular oxygen (O_2) are included, mainly superoxide anion (O^{2-}), hydrogen peroxide (H_2O_2), and hydroxyl radical (OH^-), all of which are highly reactive and capable of causing damage in the cell. These reactive species can be generated naturally by exhibiting a relevant function in cell biology or by inducing oxidizing agents in the medium [34].

Oxidative stress in the cell is caused by an imbalance between the production of ROS and the ability of the system to detoxify them or repair the resulting damage [35]. In the lungs, a particular target of PM, oxidative stress initiates the synthesis of mediators of pulmonary inflammation in lung epithelial cells triggering the activation of carcinogenic mechanisms (**Figure 1**). Inflammatory cells are particularly effective in generating most of the ROS. The activation of the redox metabolism of inflammatory cells generates a highly oxidative environment within an organ for aerobic organisms. ROS-mediated inflammation teams with another type of chemical species such as reactive nitrogen species (RNS) which also causes oxidative damage to cellular components. Many proinflammatory mediators, especially cytokines, chemokines, and prostaglandins, turn on the angiogenesis switches mainly

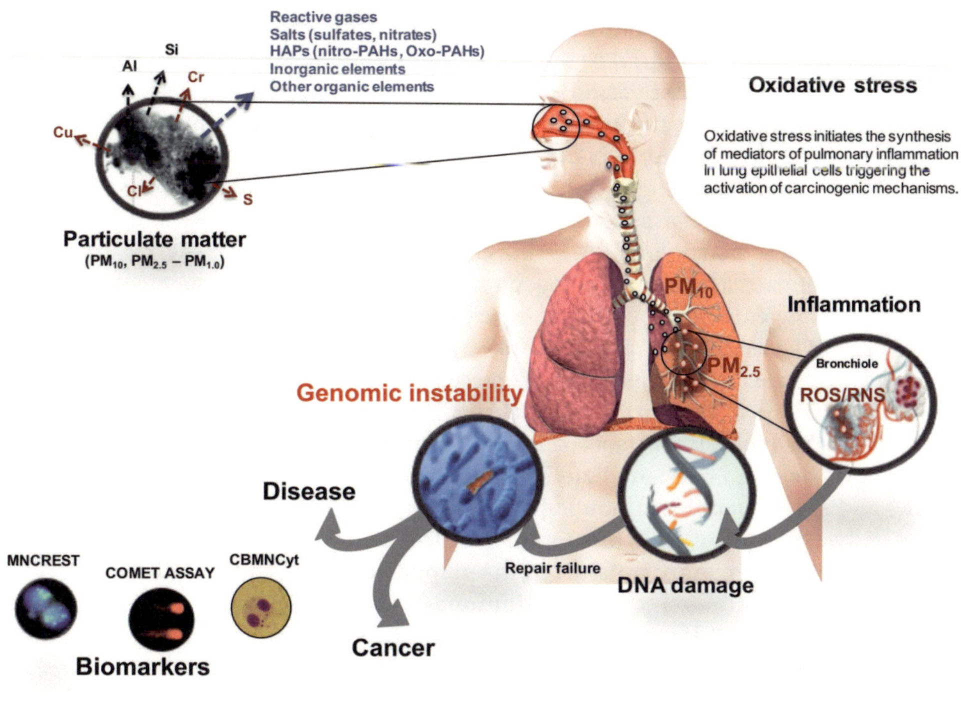

Figure 1.
Main processes and biomarkers associated with genomic instability, inflammation and cancer risk induced by particulate matter exposure.

controlled by vascular endothelial growth factors [36, 37]. The possible mechanisms by which inflammation can contribute to carcinogenesis include genomic instability, alterations in epigenetic events and subsequent inappropriate gene expression, enhanced proliferation of initiated cells, resistance to apoptosis, aggressive tumor neovascularization, invasion through the tumor-associated basement membrane, angiogenesis, and metastasis [36].

Oxidative damage generated by both ROS and RNS species in DNA is considered one of the most harmful effects for the cell since they can produce irreversible changes in the genome. Chemical modifications in DNA structure include strand breaks, sugar moiety modification, nitrogenous base oxidation, and generation of apurinic/apyrimidinic sites (AP sites) [38]. This type of DNA damage can be generated with frequencies between 104 and 105 DNA mutations per cell/day. This DNA damage can also produce several chromosomal alterations such as deletions, insertions, or translocations increasing the toxic spectrum for the cell. Accumulation of these genomic alterations may cause dysregulation of cell division, the imbalance between cell growth and death, and cancer [18].

The use of biological monitoring procedures, or biomonitoring, through specific biomarkers can assess the effects of PM exposure and its possible impact on the organism. Early biomonitoring allows detection of the first alterations during the non-malignant phase, including the measurable changes (biochemical, physiological, or morphological) that associate a toxic exposure with any early biochemical alteration.

3.1 Molecular mechanisms associate with genomic instability and cancer by PM exposure

The International Agency for Research on Cancer (IARC) has classified exposure to PM in air pollution as a human carcinogen [2]. The molecular reactions induced by the PM exposure are often initiated by reactive PM constituents including metals and various PAHs and PAH's derivatives like nitro-PAHs and various oxo-PAHs (quinones). These substances are potent oxidants, either through direct effects on proteins, lipids, mitochondrial or nuclear DNA or indirectly through the generation of free radicals and activation of intracellular oxidant pathways [11, 39]. Correspondingly, several studies have shown that other transition metals (Fe, Cu, Cr, and V) with catalytic activity during Fenton's reaction ($Fe^{2+} + H_2O_2 + H^+ \rightarrow Fe^{3+} + OH^{\cdot} + H_2O$) generate the highly reactive hydroxyl radical able to induce oxidative DNA damage, oxidative stress, and inflammatory responses [11].

Depending on its structure, PAHs show carcinogenic potential. IARC classifies these compounds as a human carcinogen (group 1), probably carcinogenic (group 2A), possibly carcinogenic (group 2B), and not classified as carcinogenic (group 3). Particularly, The HAPs that have angulated structures typically react with adenine residues and are related to a higher carcinogenic activity compared to those with a linear and more condensed structure, which usually react with guanine residues [40].

Many of the biological effects of PAHs, including oxidative stress and DNA damage, are believed to be mediated by activation of the aryl hydrocarbon receptor (AhR) and subsequent induction metabolism by cytochrome P450 (CYP) enzymes [41–43]. The binding of PAH metabolites to DNA and the associated effects that occur as a consequence are considered the main mechanisms of mutagenicity and carcinogenicity attributed to PAHs. Additionally, it is believed that the formation of redox-active quinones is catalyzed by dihydrodiol dehydrogenases, also contributing to PAH carcinogenesis and tumor promotion [44].

At least three distinct molecular mechanisms have been proposed to explain the process of tumor initiation by exposure to PAHs. These models include the formation of (1) diol-epoxide, (2) radical cations, and (3) o-quinones. The metabolism of PAHs into diol-epoxide may lead to the formation of DNA adducts, mainly in guanines and adenines, generating mutations in proto-oncogenes and tumor suppressor genes. The radical cation leads to the formation of adducts of DNA, generating AP sites. Finally, o-quinones can generate ROS and potentially cause mutations in TP53 and other tumor suppressor genes and/or proto-oncogenes [45].

On the other hand, oxy- and nitro-PAHs, which consist of oxygen and nitrogen derivatives of PAHs, respectively, play an important role in the mutagenicity attributed to PM. Studies with *Salmonella* strains (YG1041) sensitive to this group of organic compounds indicated a mutagenic activity for a fraction of nitro-PAHs, whereas oxy-PAHs can generate DNA adducts [46].

Besides, transition metal ions with redox potential, which are presented in PM (adsorbed at high concentrations inside particle cavities), can contribute to ROS overproduction and play an important role in oxidative DNA and protein damage [47]. Soluble metals on inhaled particles, such as Fe, Ni, V, Co, Cu, and Cr, were associated with increased ROS production, followed by cellular oxidative stress in airway epithelial cells [48]. Studies have identified certain metals as responsible for oxidant effects and inflammation in experimental animals, by using diverse metal chelators (such as EDTA, which increase the redox reactivity of some metals) and antioxidants (which scavenge oxygen-free radicals) for metal assessment [44].

The different types of particles in PM, their extracts, as well as single obtained components, all have demonstrated genotoxic effects in human and animal studies both in vivo and in vitro [23]. Several studies have shown that cells may be arrested in various parts of the cell cycle [49, 50]. Most often, such effects have been linked to DNA damage, and following PM exposure, this DNA damage includes mainly DNA single-strand breaks, alkali-labile single-strand DNA breaks, and various forms of oxidative DNA damage including oxidized guanines measured as 8-oxo-7,8-dihydroguanine (8-oxoGua) adducts and lesions detected as formamidopyrimidine DNA glycosylase (FPG) sites by the comet assay [51]. Often this type of damage is associated with chromosomal damage induction. These biomarkers are used to assess genotoxic effects on human populations exposed to complex mixtures of chemicals.

3.2 Risk biomarkers based on the determination of genomic instability for estimation of cancer risk

Exposure biomarkers reflect human exposure on different routes. Biological monitoring of PAHs is restricted because of the few PAHs for which metabolites are available as standards. However, this limitation is partially overcome by the use of metabolite markers of total exposure to PAHs, such as 1-hydroxypyrene (1-OHP) [48, 52]. Several studies have shown that urinary 1-OHP is a useful biomarker of both environmental and occupational exposures to PAHs and shows a correlation with genotoxic effect biomarkers measured in peripheral blood lymphocytes [53, 54].

In addition to these biochemical markers, other cytogenetic biomarkers have been suggested for the identification of cancer risk; the most generalized and best-characterized biomarker for evaluating the mutagenic effects and possible cancer risk in populations exposed to PM is the assessment of micronuclei (MN) frequency in vivo. MN is an effect biomarker consisting of small nuclear masses of genetic material separate from the main nucleus and arising in the dividing cells. They are measured 1/3 to 1/16 of the size of the nucleus and are delimited by a nuclear membrane. MNs are derived from chromosomal breaks (clastogenic origin) and/or whole chromosomes (aneugenic origin). MN composed of fragments of chromosomes (clastogenic) can result from the direct breaking of the double strand of DNA, conversion from single-stranded to double-stranded strand after cell replication or inhibition of DNA synthesis. The MN formed by whole chromosomes (aneugenic) is mainly caused by defects in the mechanism of chromosomal segregation, such as deficiencies in the control of cell cycle genes, mitotic spindle faults, kinetochore, or other parts of the mitotic apparatus, mechanical rupture, or hypomethylation of centromeric DNA [55–58]. For MN assessment the used protocol is the cytokinesis-block cytome micronucleus assay (CBMNCyt), whereas for rapid chromosomal break evaluation, the micronucleus assay with CREST immunostaining (MNCREST) is often used.

CBMNCyt used in primary cultured cells such as lymphocytes allows measuring not only genotoxicity parameters (solely MN frequency) but also cytokinesis defects (binucleate cells) and includes MNBN (MN in binucleated or cytokinesis blocked cells), a biomarker of chromosome breakage and/or whole chromosome loss; MNMONO (MN in mononucleated cells), a biomarker of chromosomal damage induced and expressed in vivo before the start of the CBMN assay culture; NPBs (nucleoplasmic bridges), a biomarker of DNA misrepair and/or telomere end-fusions; and NBUDs (or "nuclear buds"), a biomarker of elimination of amplified DNA and/or DNA repair complexes [55]. In addition, the assay allows measuring the proliferative potential (basal cells) and various forms of cell death (pyknotic, karyolytic, karyorrhexis, and chromatin condensation). So, the application of this approach provides information on genotoxic, cytotoxic, and cytostatic effects increasing the predictive capacity of the bioassay [59]. However, it is worth emphasizing that only the frequency of MN has been associated with an increased risk of cancer development, neurodegenerative diseases, and acceleration of aging [56, 60]. MNMONO frequencies may give an estimation of the genome instability accumulated over many years in stem cells and circulating T lymphocytes long before the blood was sampled, whereas MNBN cells provide an additional measure of lesions that have accumulated in DNA or key proteins [61].

In a study developed by our laboratory, we assessed PM exposure in populations with residential proximity to open-pit coal mine in Northern Colombia and investigated the correlation between chromosomal damage and genetic instability evaluated by CBMNcyt in isolated lymphocytes of individuals with residential proximity to the coal mining corridor and its relation with measured PM_{10} and $PM_{2,5}$ levels. Our results revealed a significant increase in MNBN and MNMONO cells in individuals with residential proximity to open-pit coal mines. Additionally, correlation analysis demonstrated a highly significant association between $PM_{2.5}$ levels, MNBN frequencies, and CREST+ micronucleus induction in exposed residents. These results suggest that $PM_{2.5}$ fraction generated in coal mining activities may induce whole chromosome loss (aneuploidy) preferentially, although there are also chromosome breaks. This aneugenic effect may be associated with an oxidative stress status inside the cell, potentially capable of causing mitotic arrest (elevated MNMONO frequency), centromere damage, kinetochore malfunction, or disruption of the mitotic spindle [18].

Other types of MN assessment use exfoliated buccal cells isolated from exposed individuals. The micronucleus test in oral mucosal cells or buccal MN cytome assay (BMCyt) has been widely used in studies of populations exposed environmentally or occupationally to genotoxic agents. Previous work from our laboratory demonstrated MN formation in exfoliated buccal cells of workers occupationally exposed to open coal mining residues, which correlated with PM increased levels detected by BMCyt assay [62]. This technique is particularly attractive because oral mucosal cells can be collected in a minimally invasive manner [63, 64].

4. Conclusions

Sufficient evidence has been accumulated from epidemiological studies that support the fact that a broad spectrum of health outcome variables may come from short-term exposure to coarse, fine, and ultrafine PM. This association is consistent with experimental evidence that identifies different mechanisms of damage at a cellular level: inflammation, oxidative stress, cytotoxicity, alterations of autonomic nervous system, and coagulation. In relation to chronic effects on health, studies are less numerous, and the evidence is still inconsistent. Previous work suggests that PM exerts its genotoxic and carcinogenic effects through the generation of DNA damage and chromosomal instability. The biological mechanisms behind these associations are not fully understood, but toxicological results in vitro have shown that PM induces several types of adverse cellular effects.

Author details

Lyda Espitia-Pérez*, Luisa Jiménez-Vidal and Pedro Espitia-Pérez
Grupo de Investigaciones Biomedicas y Biología Molecular, Universidad del Sinú, Montería, Córdoba, Colombia

*Address all correspondence to: lydaespitia@unisinu.edu.co

References

[1] Prüss-Üstün A, Corvalán C. Preventing disease through healthy environments: A global assessment of the burden of disease from environmental risks. Geneva: World Health Organization; 2016

[2] Loomis D, Grosse Y, Lauby-Secretan B, Ghissassi FE, Bouvard V, Benbrahim-Tallaa L, et al. The carcinogenicity of outdoor air pollution. The Lancet Oncology. 2013;**14**(13):1262-1263

[3] EPA USEPA. Executive summary. In: Air Quality Criteria for Particulate Matter. Vol. I. Publication No. EPA/600/P-95/001/aF; National Center for Environmental Assessment; Research Triangle Park. 1996. pp. 1-21

[4] Andreau K, Leroux M, Bouharrour A. Health and cellular impacts of air pollutants: From cytoprotection to cytotoxicity. Biochemistry Research International. 2012;**2012**:1-18

[5] Pope CA 3rd, Burnett RT, Thun MJ, Calle EE, Krewski D, Ito K, et al. Lung cancer, cardiopulmonary mortality, and long-term exposure to fine particulate air pollution. Journal of the American Medical Association. 2002;**287**(9):1132-1141

[6] Santibáñez-Andrade M, Quezada-Maldonado EM, Osornio-Vargas Á, Sánchez-Pérez Y, García-Cuellar CM. Air pollution and genomic instability: The role of particulate matter in lung carcinogenesis. Environmental Pollution. 2017;**229**:412-422

[7] Broustas CG, Lieberman HB. DNA damage response genes and the development of cancer metastasis. Radiation Research. 2014;**181**(2):111-130

[8] Benford D, Hanley B, Bottrill K, Oehlschlager S, Balls M, Branca F, et al. Biomarkers as predictive tools in toxicity testing. Alternatives to Laboratory Animals. 2000;**28**:119-131

[9] Hu Z, Brooks SA, Dormoy V, Hsu CW, Hsu HY, Lin LT, et al. Assessing the carcinogenic potential of low-dose exposures to chemical mixtures in the environment: Focus on the cancer hallmark of tumor angiogenesis. Carcinogenesis. 2015;**36**(Suppl 1): S184-S202

[10] Vallero D. Air pollution decision tools. In: Fundamentals of Air Pollution. 5th ed. Amsterdam: Academic Press; 2014. pp. 83-109

[11] Lodovici M, Bigagli E. Oxidative stress and air pollution exposure. Journal of Toxicology. 2011;**2011**:1-9

[12] Grantz DA, Garner JHB, Johnson DW. Ecological effects of particulate matter. Environment International. 2003;**29**(2-3):213-239

[13] Pey J, Rodríguez S, Querol X, Alastuey A, Moreno T, Putaud JP, et al. Variations of urban aerosols in the western mediterranean. Atmospheric Environment. 2008;**42**(40):9052-9062

[14] Zheng N, Liu J, Wang Q, Liang Z. Health risk assessment of heavy metal exposure to street dust in the zinc smelting district, northeast of China. Science of the Total Environment. 2010;**408**(4):726-733

[15] Zhou S, Yuan Q, Li W, Lu Y, Zhang Y, Wang W. Trace metals in atmospheric fine particles in one industrial urban city: Spatial variations, sources, and health implications. Journal of Environmental Sciences. 2014;**26**(1):205-213

[16] Johansson C, Norman M, Burman L. Road traffic emission factors for heavy metals. Atmospheric Environment. 2009;**43**(31):4681-4688

[17] Lough GC, Schauer JJ, Park JS, Shafer MM, Deminter JT, Weinstein JP. Emissions of metals associated

with motor vehicle roadways. Environmental Science & Technology. 2005;**39**(3):826-836

[18] Espitia-Perez L, da Silva J, Espitia-Perez P, Brango H, Salcedo-Arteaga S, Hoyos-Giraldo LS, et al. Cytogenetic instability in populations with residential proximity to open-pit coal mine in northern Colombia in relation to PM10 and PM2. 5 levels. Ecotoxicology and Environmental Safety. 2018;**148**:453-466

[19] Campagna M, Pilia I, Marcias G, Frattolillo A, Pili S, Bernabei M, et al. Ultrafine particle distribution and chemical composition assessment during military operative trainings. International Journal of Environmental Research and Public Health. 2017;**14**(6):579

[20] Lu F, Xu D, Cheng Y, Dong S, Guo C, Jiang X, et al. Systematic review and meta-analysis of the adverse health effects of ambient PM2.5 and PM10 pollution in the Chinese population. Environmental Research. 2015;**136**:196-204

[21] Baldauf R, Devlin R, Gehr P, Giannelli R, Hassett-Sipple B, Jung H, et al. Ultrafine particle metrics and research considerations: Review of the 2015 UFP workshop. International Journal of Environmental Research and Public Health. 2016;**13**(11):1054

[22] Cheng H, Gong W, Wang Z, Zhang F, Wang X, Lv X, et al. Ionic composition of submicron particles (PM1.0) during the long-lasting haze period in January 2013 in Wuhan, Central China. Journal of Environmental Sciences. 2014;**26**(4):810-817

[23] Nemmar A, Holme JA, Rosas I, Schwarze PE, Alfaro-Moreno E. Recent advances in particulate matter and nanoparticle toxicology: A review of the *in vivo* and *in vitro* studies. BioMed Research International. 2013;**2013**:279371

[24] Kawanaka Y, Matsumoto E, Sakamoto K, Wang N, Yun S-J. Size distributions of mutagenic compounds and mutagenicity in atmospheric particulate matter collected with a low-pressure cascade impactor. Atmospheric Environment. 2004;**38**(14):2125-2132

[25] Araujo JA, Nel AE. Particulate matter and atherosclerosis: Role of particle size, composition and oxidative stress. Particle and Fibre Toxicology. 2009;**6**:24

[26] Weichenthal SA, Godri-Pollitt K, Villeneuve PJ. PM2.5, oxidant defence and cardiorespiratory health: A review. Environmental Health. 2013;**12**:40

[27] Kurth L, Kolker A, Engle M, Geboy N, Hendryx M, Orem W, et al. Atmospheric particulate matter in proximity to mountaintop coal mines: Sources and potential environmental and human health impacts. Environmental Geochemistry and Health. 2015;**37**(3):529-544

[28] Brook RD, Rajagopalan S, Pope CA 3rd, Brook JR, Bhatnagar A, Diez-Roux AV, et al. Particulate matter air pollution and cardiovascular disease: An update to the scientific statement from the American Heart Association. Circulation. 2010;**121**(21):2331-2378

[29] Achilleos S, Kioumourtzoglou MA, Wu CD, Schwartz JD, Koutrakis P, Papatheodorou SI. Acute effects of fine particulate matter constituents on mortality: A systematic review and meta-regression analysis. Environment International. 2017;**109**:89-100

[30] Morales-Suarez-Varela M, Peraita-Costa I, Llopis-Gonzalez A. Systematic review of the association between particulate matter exposure and autism spectrum disorders. Environmental Research. 2017;**153**:150-160

[31] Weinmayr G, Hennig F, Fuks K, Nonnemacher M, Jakobs H, Mohlenkamp S, et al. Long-term exposure to fine particulate matter and incidence of type 2 diabetes mellitus in a cohort study: Effects of total and traffic-specific air pollution. Environmental Health. 2015;**14**:53

[32] Heusinkveld HJ, Wahle T, Campbell A, Westerink RHS, Tran L, Johnston H, et al. Neurodegenerative and neurological disorders by small inhaled particles. Neurotoxicology. 2016;**56**:94-106

[33] Li N, Xia T, Nel AE. The role of oxidative stress in ambient particulate matter-induced lung diseases and its implications in the toxicity of engineered nanoparticles. Free Radical Biology & Medicine. 2008;**44**(9):1689-1699

[34] Juan ER. Papel del Estrés Oxidativo Sobre la Estabilidad Genética y la Bioseguridad de las Células Madre Mesenquimales Humanas Adultas. Universidad Autónoma de Madrid; 2012

[35] Griendling KK, FitzGerald GA. Oxidative stress and cardiovascular injury. Circulation. 2003;**108**(16):1912-1916

[36] Valavanidis A, Vlachogianni T, Fiotakis K, Loridas S. Pulmonary oxidative stress, inflammation and cancer: Respirable particulate matter, fibrous dusts and ozone as major causes of lung carcinogenesis through reactive oxygen species mechanisms. International Journal of Environmental Research and Public Health. 2013;**10**(9):3886-3907

[37] Costa C, Incio J, Soares R. Angiogenesis and chronic inflammation: Cause or consequence? Angiogenesis. 2007;**10**(3):149-166

[38] Gajewski TF, Schreiber H, Fu YX. Innate and adaptive immune cells in the tumor microenvironment. Nature Immunology. 2013;**14**(10):1014-1022

[39] Moller P, Loft S. Oxidative damage to DNA and lipids as biomarkers of exposure to air pollution. Environmental Health Perspectives. 2010;**118**(8):1126-1136

[40] Galvão DO. Avaliação do Potencial Genotóxico e Citotóxico Associado a Queima Artesanal da Castanha de Caju. Universidade Federal do Rio Grande do Norte; 2011

[41] Jarvis IW, Dreij K, Mattsson A, Jernstrom B, Stenius U. Interactions between polycyclic aromatic hydrocarbons in complex mixtures and implications for cancer risk assessment. Toxicology. 2014;**321**:27-39

[42] Jarvis IW, Bergvall C, Bottai M, Westerholm R, Stenius U, Dreij K. Persistent activation of DNA damage signaling in response to complex mixtures of PAHs in air particulate matter. Toxicology and Applied Pharmacology. 2013;**266**(3):408-418

[43] Murray IA, Patterson AD, Perdew GH. Aryl hydrocarbon receptor ligands in cancer friend and foe. Nature Reviews. Cancer. 2014;**14**(12):801-814

[44] Valavanidis A, Fiotakis K, Vlachogianni T. Airborne particulate matter and human health: Toxicological assessment and importance of size and composition of particles for oxidative damage and carcinogenic mechanisms. Journal of Environmental Science and Health Part C Environmental Carcinogenesis & Ecotoxicology Reviews. 2008;**26**(4):339-362

[45] EPA. Development of a Relative Potency Factor (RPF) Approach for Polycyclic Aromatic Hydrocarbon (PAH) Mixtures. 2010

[46] Umbuzeiro GA, Franco A, Martins MH, Kummrow F, Carvalho L, Schmeiser HH, et al. Mutagenicity and DNA adduct formation of PAH, nitro-PAH, and oxy-PAH fractions of

atmospheric particulate matter from Sao Paulo, Brazil. Mutation Research. 2008;**652**(1):72-80

[47] Valko M, Rhodes CJ, Moncol J, Izakovic M, Mazur M. Free radicals, metals and antioxidants in oxidative stress-induced cancer. Chemico-Biological Interactions. 2006;**160**(1):1-40

[48] Yuan TH, Shie RH, Chin YY, Chan CC. Assessment of the levels of urinary 1-hydroxypyrene and air polycyclic aromatic hydrocarbon in PM2.5 for adult exposure to the petrochemical complex emissions. Environmental Research. 2015;**136**:219-226

[49] Gualtieri M, Ovrevik J, Mollerup S, Asare N, Longhin E, Dahlman HJ, et al. Airborne urban particles (Milan winter-PM2.5) cause mitotic arrest and cell death: Effects on DNA, mitochondria, AhR binding and spindle organization. Mutation Research. 2011;**713**(1-2):18-31

[50] Danielsen PH, Loft S, Kocbach A, Schwarze PE, Moller P. Oxidative damage to DNA and repair induced by Norwegian wood smoke particles in human A549 and THP-1 cell lines. Mutation Research. 2009;**674**(1-2):116-122

[51] Dubinett SM, Lee JM, Sharma S, Mule JJ. Chemokines: Can effector cells be redirected to the site of the tumor? Cancer Journal. 2010;**16**(4):325-335

[52] Hansen AM, Mathiesen L, Pedersen M, Knudsen LE. Urinary 1-hydroxypyrene (1-HP) in environmental and occupational studies—A review. International Journal of Hygiene and Environmental Health. 2008;**211**(5-6):471-503

[53] Duan H, Leng S, Pan Z, Dai Y, Niu Y, Huang C, et al. Biomarkers measured by cytokinesis-block micronucleus cytome assay for evaluating genetic damages induced by polycyclic aromatic hydrocarbons. Mutation Research. 2009;**677**(1-2):93-99

[54] Leng S, Dai Y, Niu Y, Pan Z, Li X, Cheng J, et al. Effects of genetic polymorphisms of metabolic enzymes on cytokinesis-block micronucleus in peripheral blood lymphoc. Cancer Epidemiology, Biomarkers & Prevention. 2004;**13**(10):1631-1639

[55] Fenech M. Cytokinesis-block micronucleus assay evolves into a "cytome" assay of chromosomal instability, mitotic dysfunction and cell death. Mutation Research. 2006;**600**(1-2):58-66

[56] Bolognesi C, Knasmueller S, Nersesyan A, Thomas P, Fenech M. The HUMNxl scoring criteria for different cell types and nuclear anomalies in the buccal micronucleus cytome assay—An update and expanded photogallery. Mutation Research. 2013;**753**(2):100-113

[57] Terradas M, Martin M, Genesca A. Impaired nuclear functions in micronuclei results in genome instability and chromothripsis. Archives of Toxicology. 2016;**90**(11):2657-2667

[58] Iarmarcovai G, Botta A, Orsiere T. Number of centromeric signals in micronuclei and mechanisms of aneuploidy. Toxicology Letters. 2006;**166**(1):1-10

[59] Bolognesi C, Bonassi S, Knasmueller S, Fenech M, Bruzzone M, Lando C, et al. Clinical application of micronucleus test in exfoliated buccal cells: A systematic review and metanalysis. Mutation Research, Reviews in Mutation Research. 2015;**766**:20-31

[60] Bonassi S, Znaor A, Ceppi M, Lando C, Chang WP, Holland N, et al. An increased micronucleus frequency in peripheral blood lymphocytes

predicts the risk of cancer in humans. Carcinogenesis. 2007;**28**(3):625-631

[61] Kirsch-Voldersa M, Bonassi S, Knasmueller S, Holland N, Bolognesi C, Fenech FM. Commentary critical questions, misconceptions and a road map for improving the use of the lymphocyte cytokinesis-block micronucleus assay for *in vivo* biomonitoring of human exposure to genotoxic chemicals—A HUMN project perspective. Mutation Research. 2014;**759**:49-58

[62] Leon-Mejia G, Quintana M, Debastiani R, Dias J, Espitia-Perez L, Hartmann A, et al. Genetic damage in coal miners evaluated by buccal micronucleus cytome assay. Ecotoxicology and Environmental Safety. 2014;**107**:133-139

[63] Thomas P, Holland N, Bolognesi C, Kirsch-Volders M, Bonassi S, Zeiger E, et al. Buccal micronucleus cytome assay. Nature Protocols. 2009;**4**(6):825-837

[64] Doherty A, Steven MB, Jeffrey C. Bemis. The in vitro micronucleus assay. Genetic Toxicology Testing. Academic Press; 2016. pp. 161-205

Chapter 2

Pollution of Water Resources and Environmental Impacts in Urban Areas of Developing Countries: Case of the City of Les Cayes (Haiti)

Ketty Balthazard-Accou, Evens Emmanuel, Patrice Agnamey and Christian Raccurt

Abstract

Many cities in developing countries are facing serious problems of microbiological quality of their water resources. In this context, chlorination is used as common method of treating water intended for human consumption. However, it has been shown that disinfection by chlorination is ineffective in inactivating *Cryptosporidium* oocysts. Therefore, the physicochemical behavior of *Cryptosporidium* oocysts and geological formation of those areas become an important environmental issue of research. In Haiti, *Cryptosporidium* oocysts have been identified in the groundwater being used for human consumption in Les Cayes. Moreover, cryptosporidiosis is one of the most frequent causes of diarrhea in Haiti. The transfer of *Cryptosporidium* oocysts, through an alluvial formation from Les Cayes (Haiti), was investigated. The aim of this chapter was (i) to review the biological cycle of *Cryptosporidium* and the physicochemical behavior of *Cryptosporidium* oocysts in order (ii) to understand their movement through soils and (iii) to evaluate the chemical conditions and soil characteristics which can constitute factors influencing the retention of oocysts or facilitate their transfer into groundwater.

Keywords: *Cryptosporidium* oocyst, soil, transfer, pollution, groundwater resources, Les Cayes (Haiti)

1. Introduction

Pollution of water resources has become a major environmental challenge for many urban areas in both developed and developing countries [1–3]. Although developing countries are characterized by a lower industrialization, the deficiency observed in solid waste and wastewater management and the lack of city planning constitute factors facilitating the environmental pollution of cities. Moreover, unexpected population growth is related to water quality degradation and is causing large increase in nutrients and microbial loads [4–6]. Therefore, urban areas have the potential that generate environmental impacts at multiple scales [4].

Urbanization often causes environmental degradation and harms human health particularly in developing countries [7].

Due to reasons relating to the economic problems of developing countries, when urban effluents are actually collected, they are most usually discharged into open drainage canals or into septic tanks equipped with infiltration shafts [8]. Infiltration of urban stormwater runoff can be also considered as one of the main factors of the deterioration of soils and groundwater quality [3]. This last is increasingly subject to intensive voluntary discharges of highly polluted effluents, wastewater, and runoff water in urban areas [9]. Studies have shown that in developing countries there is a strong likelihood of a marked correlation between the groundwater contamination in urban areas and the way in which public services operate [10]. In the specific socioeconomical context of developing countries, there is an important challenge of public health related to the possibility of the appearance of biological risk due to the contamination of groundwater resources by pathogenic microorganisms.

In Haiti, oocysts of *Cryptosporidium* have been detected in surface water used as drinking water and in the water supplied by the public water service of Port-au-Prince [11, 12]. In the surrounding region of Cap-Haitien, investigations conducted on water resources revealed the presence of *Cryptosporidium* oocysts in surface and groundwater used by the population for domestic purposes [13, 14]. The number of oocysts detected in the city of Cap-Haitien ranges from 741 to 6088 oocysts per 100 liters of water.

In the city Les Cayes (Haiti) has highlighted the presence of the *Cryptosporidium* oocyst groundwater used by the population for domestic purposes [10, 15, 16]. The number of oocysts detected varied from 5 to 100 per 100 l of water [15]. These results show that the surface water and groundwater of Cayes are contaminated by pollution of fecal origin and are a source of potential biological risk for the health of the population exposed. Human risk assessment due to these results shows in evidence biological risks for consumers that range from 4 to 1274 oocysts per 100 l of water. The management phase of this assessment allows for the questioning of physicochemical mechanisms governing the transfer of oocysts from the ground to underground waters. The objective of this study was to investigate the behavior of *Cryptosporidium* oocysts under physicochemical conditions and soil characteristics in saturated porous media of Les Cayes and to describe the water pollution dynamics of *Cryptosporidium* oocysts.

This work reported in this chapter has four main sections. Initially, we introduce the chapter. The first section proposes a synthesis of information on the biological cycle of *Cryptosporidium*, followed by a review of source and transport of the physicochemical behavior of *Cryptosporidium* oocysts. The second section describes the geography of the City of Les Cayes. It also describes the hydrogeological properties of this city while taking care to underline the management system of wastewater and solid waste developed in that area. The third section presents the chemical conditions and soil characteristics which can constitute factors influencing the retention of oocysts or facilitate their transfer into groundwater. The fourth section is devoted also to sharing results of works on the mobility and retention of *C. parvum* oocysts in soil of the City of Les Cayes.

2. Life cycle of *Cryptosporidium*

2.1 Biological cycle of *Cryptosporidium*

Cryptosporidium represents the genus of a variety of intracellular parasites that infect vertebrates, including humans, worldwide. *Cryptosporidium* belongs

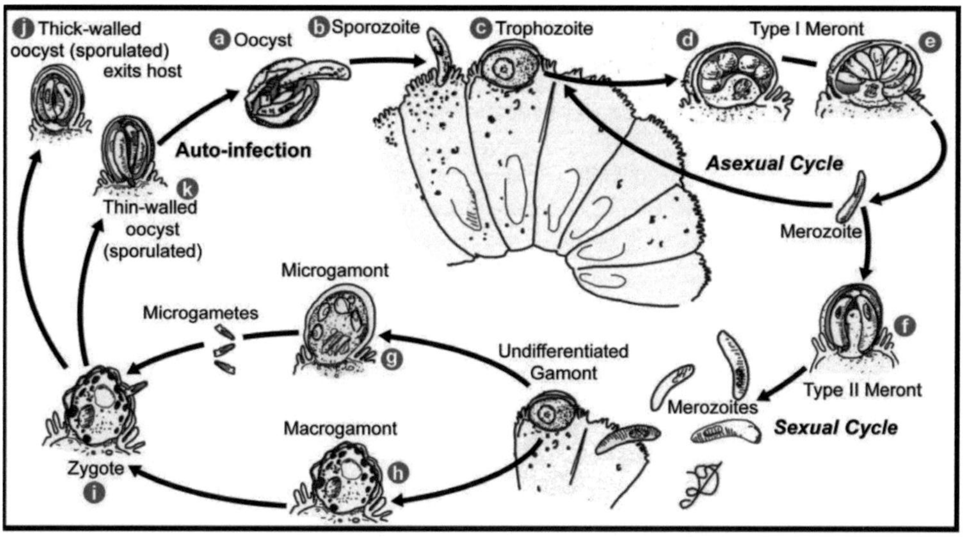

Figure 1.
Life cycle of Cryptosporidium. Reported in [10]. Source: http://www.stanford.edu/group/parasites/ParaSites2005/Cryptosporidiosis/index.html.

to Apicomplexa (synonym Sporozoa), an obligate parasitic group of eukaryotes. However, recent studies, based on genetics and physiology, have now relocated the genus *Cryptosporidium* from Coccidia to *Gregarina*, which includes free-living stages, enabling host-free multiplication, and so may constitute an additional risk factor for human infection [17]. The life cycle of *Cryptosporidium* is monoxenous, which means that every stage in the parasitic cycle's development takes place inside the same host. The multiplication cycle comprises of sexual and asexual stages. The progress of this cycle is schematically depicted in **Figure 1**. The asexual multiplication results in merozoite formation, enabling reinfection of intestinal epithelial cells and the sexual cycle culminating in thin or thick-walled sporozoite-containing oocysts (4–6 μm with an ovoidal or round shape) [18]. Infection occurs when the oocysts are ingested by a suitable host. While in the intestines, the oocyst releases sporozoites which invade the epithelial linings of the intestines or the lungs. The infectious oocysts are passed through the feces and enter the environment. Under natural conditions, fecal matter shelters oocysts from desiccation and increases the impermeability of the wall to small molecules, thereby reducing their exposure to lethal environmental factors [19]. The resistance of oocysts in a solid matrix such as soil has become a crucial parameter in understanding their transfer to lower layers. Oocysts persist longer in soil than in water at the same temperature, with a preference for moist silty soils rather than moist clay or sandy [20]. Oocysts can remain viable and infectious in water for several months at temperatures ranging from 0 to 30°C. Other tests have shown that boiling water can kill *Cryptosporidium* oocysts in less than a minute [21]. The exposure to sunlight had no effect on the viability of *Cryptosporidium* oocysts, but UV at 265 nm and black light at 365 nm lead to a reduction in the number of viable oocysts [22].

2.2 Source and transport of *Cryptosporidium parvum* oocysts through soils

Cryptosporidium is a zoonotic intestinal protozoan parasite that affects the gastrointestinal tract of humans and animals [23, 24]. This protozoan parasite is transmitted via the fecal-oral route and is an important cause of childhood diarrhea and mortality [25]. In developing countries, 8–19% of diarreal diseases are attributed to

Cryptosporidium [26]. Furthermore, 10% of the population in developing countries excretes oocysts which the scattering and resistant form of *Cryptosporidium* sp. is eliminated with feces [27]. Immunocompetent persons will usually recover from the illness within 2 weeks, whereas immunocompromised individuals, including patients undergoing chemotherapy for cancer, patients with AIDS, infants, children, and elderly, may be afflicted with chronic and debilitating illness [28]. In natural surface water and soil, *Cryptosporidium* oocysts can survive up to 6 months [19, 29]. Oocysts are resistant to a number of environmental stresses, including chlorination during drinking water treatment.

The infectivity oocysts are high, and ingestion of just a single oocyst generates an infection probability [30]. Many outbreaks of foodborne cryptosporidiosis have been described also. In Milwaukee in North America (1993), a massive outbreak of acute diarrhea was caused by drinking water treatment deficiencies; about 403,000 persons were affected and 69 died [31]. According to [32] there have been at least 18 outbreaks of cryptosporidiosis in which foodborne transmission has been epidemiologically implicated, and 8 of these outbreaks were directly linked to consumption of fresh produce [33]. Furthermore, two more foodborne outbreaks (one in Finland and one in the UK) have been published subsequently [34, 35].

Such environmental contamination can be from soil, particularly soil amended with feces or manure, or from water such as irrigation water or wash water along the food chain [36]. Several models have been used to study pathogen transport. Previous work has investigated the transport of *Cryptosporidium* oocysts in terrestrial environments [37, 38]. To remove oocysts from water resources, several mechanisms such as filtration methods [39]; laboratory columns [40, 41] or radial stagnation point flow (RSPF) cell [42, 43] have been used. Otherwise various aspects of *C. parvum* transport and removal in granular porous media have been also examined, such as the influence of solution chemistry, fluid flow rate, and sediment grain size [40]. Detailed experimental observations have since confirmed this to be the case, especially through soil macropores and in karstic geological terrain through fractured bedrocks [44, 45]. Based on experimental evidence, it seems well established that *C. parvum* oocysts can move in soils through preferential pathways in relatively large amounts [46]. The surface properties of the oocyst wall may mediate how it survives and its interactions with chemical and particulate surfaces in the environment. Therefore, changes in the wall may affect adhesion, transport properties, and mobility in natural environments and treatment plants. Oocyst removal in porous media is still poorly understood. The transport of *Cryptosporidium* oocysts in the subsurface environment is of great concern for water quality.

2.3 Surface properties of *Cryptosporidium* oocysts

The *Cryptosporidium* oocysts are spheroidal shapes with a specific gravity of 1.0 g cm^{-3} [47]. *Cryptosporidium* oocysts' wall has three layers. An acidic glycoprotein is hypothesized to make up the outermost layer. The inner layer also appears to be a filamentous glycoprotein, while the central layer is thought to be a rigid, complex lipid [48]. The thickness of the wall and its capacity to strongly adhere to both organic and inorganic surfaces are features that could be attributed to its survival in the environment [49]. Other studies determined on the oocyst surface that it has high contents of the amino acid cysteine, proline, and histidine [50]. Otherwise oocysts have a negative surface charge under typical environmental conditions [51–57], likely due to the presence of carboxylate, carboxylic, and phosphate groups on the oocyst surface [55]. Both steric and electrostatic forces can play a role in oocyst association with suspended particles [58]. The understanding and mastering of the complex sorption phenomena involve an evaluation of the hydrophobic and electrostatic surface properties of the parasite [50]. Indeed, the surface properties of the oocyst wall may mediate how it survives and its interactions with chemical and particulate surfaces in the environment. Therefore, changes in the wall may affect adhesion, transport properties, and mobility in natural environments. The most important physical and chemical adhesion properties are the surface charge and hydrophobic characteristics [59]. The surface electrokinetic potential is negatively charged with a range from −19 to −42 mV at a neutral pH [60]. However, the negative surface charge increases with decreasing pH, and the hydrophobicity is low with high medium conductivity [48].

2.4 Transport of *Cryptosporidium* oocysts

Deyac et al. [61] elaborated in a working paper based on the data found in literature on the transport of *Cryptosporidium* oocysts. Based on its size, the *C. parvum* oocyst is physically classified as a biological colloid. Surface charges measured by the ξ potential of the oocysts have been found to be neutral to slightly negative in most natural waters. Exact values depend on analytical methods used [50, 62]. Transport and filtration of such colloids in porous media are by advection hydrodynamic dispersion and interactive processes between colloids and solids surfaces [63]. A simple one-dimensional transport model in a steady-state flow field is:

$$\frac{\partial c}{\partial t}+\frac{\rho_b \partial s}{\theta \partial t}=vd\frac{\partial^2 c}{\partial x^2}-v\left(\frac{\partial c}{\partial x}+\lambda c\right) \tag{1}$$

where c is the concentration of *C. parvum* oocysts in suspension, s is the concentration of *C. parvum* oocysts adsorbed reversibly on solid surfaces, ρ_b is bulk density, θ is porosity, d is the hydrodynamic dispersivity coefficient, v is the advective pore velocity, and λ is the colloid filtration coefficient.

It is commonly observed that v in Eq. (1) is larger for colloids than for water (velocity enhancement) [64]. Note that Eq. (1) accounts for permanent deposition (filtration) of colloids through the first-order term $v\lambda c$ as well as for reversible deposition (sorption) through the second term on the left-hand side. Several models have been introduced to describe the permanent removal of colloids by filtration onto the solid phase [65, 66]. Mass balance considerations for the deposition of colloids in a clean packed filter bed of uniform spheres yield the following relationship between the filtration coefficient and the physical properties of filter bed and colloid [66, 67]:

$$\lambda=\frac{3(1-\theta)}{2d_c}\alpha\eta \tag{2}$$

where d_c is the median grain size diameter, α is an empirical constant referred to as collision efficiency, and η is the collector efficiency. Collector efficiency, η, represents attachment to solid surfaces due to colloid advection and diffusion, interception, buoyancy, and London-van der Waals attractive forces. These four characteristics are expressed in dimensionless form by the Peclet number, N_{Pe}; the interception number, N_R; the gravitation number, N_G; and the London-van der Waals constant, N_{Lo} [66]. In addition, a correction factor, A_s, is introduced that accounts for the pore geometry and its impact on packed bed collector efficiency. Rajagopalan and Tien showed that η is then computed from [66, 67]:

$$\eta=4A_s N^{1/3}{}_{Pe}{}^{-2/3}+A_s N_{Lo} N^{1/8}{}_{R}{}^{15/8}+0.00338A_s N_G N^{1.2}{}_{R}{}^{-0.4} \tag{3}$$

For the evaluation of the *C. parvum* transport behavior in column experiments, the collector efficiency, Eq. (3) can be computed a priori from the physical properties of the pore space (porosity, median grain size, bulk density), from the physical properties of water (density, viscosity, pore velocity) and from the physical properties of the colloid (density, mean diameter, particle diffusion coefficient). The collision efficiency, α, represents an empirical constant to account for the fact that repulsive forces at the collector surface (double-layer repulsion), which are not accounted for in Eq. (3), will prevent a fraction of the colloids from attachment [65, 67].

3. Case study in the city of Les Cayes

Several studies have highlighted the presence of *Cryptosporidium* oocysts in the surface and groundwater of the coastal city of Les Cayes [10, 14, 15]. The city is located at 18°34′00″ Northern Latitude and 72°21′00″ west Longitude on the Caribbean coast, on a coastal plain with high rainfall (over 2000 mm/year). Hydrogeologically, the basin of Les Cayes includes Plaine des Cayes and its surrounding mountains. They are drained by two principal rivers: Grand Ravine of the South and l'Acul du Sud along with many other secondary rivers. The basins of these two principal rivers are not very wide (65 and 75 km^2) but benefit from a very abundant pluviometry which gives them particularly high specific outputs (70 and 55 ls/km^2). Their low water output adds up to ~2.5 m^3/s. In the case of l'Acul du Sud, this low water output is supported by an important karstic resurgence that drains the calcareous plates forming the southernmost buttresses of Massif de la Hotte's summit, Pic Macaya. Similarly, Ravine du Sud, its principal waterway, has moderate water output of 4.96 m^3/s and low water output of 1.31 m^3/s. The watershed is shared between three distinct types of aquifers: alluvial aquifers with free waters, karstic aquifers, and carbonate aquifers (fissured and fragmented), from where resurgences and outputs vary [68].

The alluvial aquifer of Plaine des Cayes is, hydrographically speaking, located in the Southwestern area of Haiti. Dominated by Massif de la Hotte which measures more than 2000 m in altitude, this area receives abundant rains at the mountaintops (more than 3000 mm/year) and gradually toward the coasts (1400 mm/year) with an average of 1900 mm/year. The renewable groundwater resources which are sustained through direct rain infiltration are concentrated in massive karstified limestones. Its aquifer constitutes, for the entire region, its most important directly exploitable underground water resource. The depth of the water table exceeds 40 m at the plain's headwaters. In the high and moderate areas, the water table is free. In the low plain, the water table is restricted under an argillaceous covering. It is supplied by abundant and direct rain infiltration (1900 mm/year) on the high and moderate areas of the plain and by discharge from the mountains caused by floods [68].

Several factors play a role in explaining the presence of *Cryptosporidium* oocysts in the groundwaters of major cities in Haiti. These same factors can also be considered to elaborate on the hypotheses relating to the contamination of the city of Les Cayes' nappe. They are (I) urban spaces of the country characterized by the absence of basic services, such that the collection and treatment of wastewater, the collection of solid waste, and the disposal of excreta and (II) the presence of latrines and septic tanks in alluvial and karstic formations and aquifers' recharge zones. This situation can contribute to the contamination of water resources originating from human fecal discharge. (III) In Haiti, the control of water quality which is to be carried out by public agencies is not always assured [69], and (IV) chlorination remains the only mode of treatment applied to raw water intended for human consumption. This is despite the fact that *Cryptosporidium* oocysts are resistant to chlorine.

4. Behavior of *Cryptosporidium* oocysts under chemical conditions in saturated porous media

The contamination of groundwater by *Cryptosporidium* oocysts has been the subject of several studies in which the authors have approached the laboratory on the behavior of *Cryptosporidium* oocysts under chemical conditions in saturated porous media. In order to appreciate the interactions between oocysts and soil (granular porous media) techniques based on the principles of colloid and surface chemistry were used.

4.1 Sources and purification of *C. parvum* oocysts

Viable *Cryptosporidium* oocysts purified using discontinuous saccharose were obtained from the National Institute of Agronomic Research (INRA). The oocysts were collected in fecal samples from naturally infected dairy calves and kept in an aqueous medium. They were stored (in the dark at 4°C) in potassium dichromate. The concentration of oocysts in the stock solution was about 2.0×10^7 oocysts/ml. They were used for laboratory experiments within 10 days of collection.

4.2 Chemical conditions

Batch equilibrium experiments were used to study the effect of chemical condition on the behavior of *Cryptosporidium* oocysts in porous media. These experiments were conducted with two electrolyte solutions: 0.003 M $CaCl_2$ and 0.001 M NaBr. The Debye-Hückel equation was used Eq. (4):

$$-log\gamma_x = \left(0.51\sqrt{I}/1 + 3.3a_x\sqrt{I}\right) \times Z_x^2 \tag{4}$$

In this equation, α_x represents the diameter of the ion nm, Z_x the charge of the ion, and the ion X is I and the ionic strength of the solution. $\alpha Ca = 0.6$; $\alpha Cl = 0.3$.

4.3 Soil composition

Five points were selected. Each point on a random sample has been taken. The samples were collected manually at a depth between 40 and 80 cm (**Figure 2**). The soil consisted of 35.6% coarse sand, 7.1% fine sands, 25.4% fine silt, 6% coarse silt, and 25.9% clay (**Table 1**). The soils were air-dried at 35°C and sieved (2 mm), which were then stored at room temperature until used. The physicochemical characteristics of soil, such as pH, organic matter, clay, and $CaCO_3$, and cation exchange capacity (CEC) were measured using standard analytical methods presented in **Table 2** and were determined at the National Laboratory of Building and Public Works (LNBTP) Laboratory Analysis of Soil Arras (INRA) and the Institute for Radiological Protection and Nuclear Safety (IRSN).

4.4 Batch experiments

In the laboratory were added 4 g of soil with a suspension of oocysts in 12 bottles of crystal polystyrene sealed at a ratio of 1:10. To avoid changing the soil properties, the ionic strength of the solutions was adjusted by the addition of a 3 mM solution of calcium chloride ($CaCl_2$) in 6 of the 12 bottle sand and a 100 mM solution of sodium bromide (NaBr) in the remaining 6. The batch tubes were placed vertically in racks on a vibration-free bench top after mixing to allow particles to settle. These were stirred for 24 h using a shaker table at 220 shakes per minute room

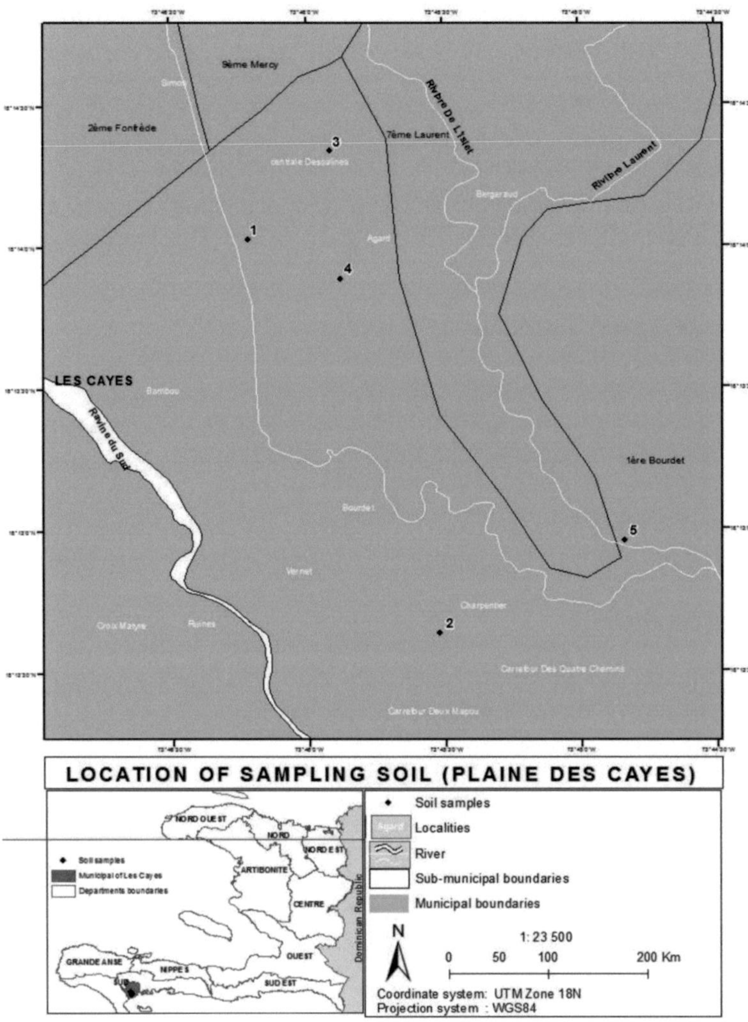

Figure 2.
Location of sampling soil (Plaine des Cayes). Source: [16].

Fraction	Particle size distribution %
Clay (< 2 µm)	25.9
Fine silt (2/20 µm)	25.4
Coarse lime (20/50 µm)	6
Fine sands (50/200 µm)	7.1
Coarse sand (200/2000 µm)	35.6

Table 1.
Particle size distribution of soil elements.

temperature (23 ± 2°C). At the end of the stirring period, the tubes were placed in an upright position for 20 h. Since soil particles settled much faster than oocysts, due to their different densities, the solution at the top of each tube was removed and

Parameters		Laboratory	Protocol excution
Sedimentometry		National Laboratory of Building and Public Works - LNBTP	NF X 31-107
Size			NF X 31-107
Water content			NF ISO 11465
Soil pH	Water-pH KCl-pH	National Institute of Agronomic Research – INRA	NF ISO 10390
Carbonate content	Total limestone Active limestone		NF ISO 10693 NF X 31-106
Organic carbon content			NF ISO 10694
Clay content			NF X 31-107
CEC			NF X 31-130
Specific soil surface		Institute for Radiological Protection and Nuclear Safety - IRSN	NF ISO 9277

Table 2.
Physicochemical analysis of soil.

analyzed for oocyst amounts. The solution was analyzed by epifluorescence, and the determination of the amount of oocysts retained in the soil (q_e) was calculated using Eq. (5):

$$q_e = (C_o - C_e) * V/m \tag{5}$$

where q_e is the amount of oocysts absorbed per unit mass of solid expressed in L/g particles; C_0, the initial concentration of suspension oocysts/L; *Ce*, the concentration of colloidal particles balanced oocysts/L; V, the volume of solution used in L; and m, the mass in grams of dry soil.

4.5 Enumeration of *C. parvum* oocysts

Enumeration of *Cryptosporidium* oocysts was conducted by the method of concentration and counting [70]. Oocyst concentration in the suspension was determined by monoclonal antibodies' staining and epifluorescence. Each final suspension tube containing oocysts was placed in an Eppendorf standard micro test tube (2 ml volume). To this suspension, a volume of 250 μl fluorescein isothiocyanate (FITC)-conjugated monoclonal antibody was added, and the mixture was incubated for 30 min at 36°C. Following incubation, the stained sample was subjected to three rinses with phosphate buffered saline (pH 7.0, 0.1 mM) and centrifugally washed (4000×*g*) for removal of unattached antibodies. Then, 100-μl aliquots were placed on six-well chamber slides and fixed with 100% methanol.

5. Retention of *C. parvum* oocysts in the soil

Tables 2 and **3** present the results of physicochemical analysis and particle size distribution of the soil of the study. These analyses indicate that the soil is characterized by fine particles; the size of the largest element is 2.50 mm.

Soil type	texture	% of soil sand	silt	clay	pH	% organic carbon	CEC (cmol/kg)[a]	Specific surface
Alluvial soil	Clay loams	42.7	31.4	25.9	8.52	10.3	15.2	16.32

[a] CEC, cation exchange capacity (units of charge per weight of soil)

Table 3.
Soil characterization data used in this study.

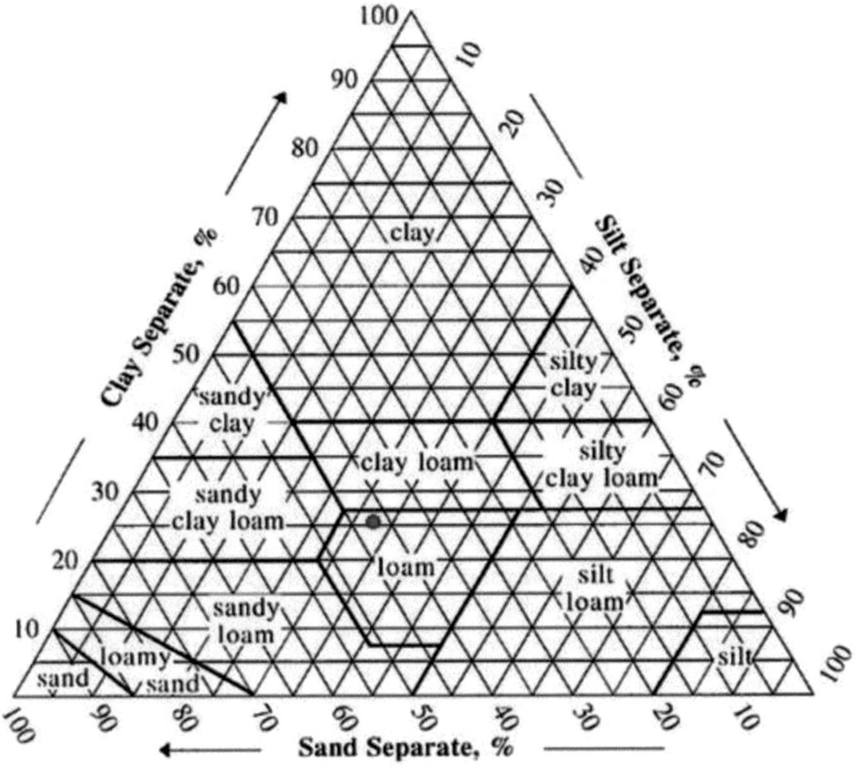

Figure 3.
Particle size distribution of the soil sample of the study. Source: [16].

This fraction represents about 25% of the sample (**Figure 3**) and consisted of 35.6% coarse sand, 7.1% fine sands, 25.4% fine silt, 6% coarse silt, and 25.9% clay. According to [71] the largest CEC values were observed for the particle size analysis 15.2 (cmol/kg) of cation exchange capacity (CEC) and a large surface area due to the presence of silts and clays there for a large number of binding sites. The highest pH value was observed pH (8.52) probably due to the high calcium carbonate content (10.3 g/kg) and a high total calcium concentration (590 g/kg).

The retention of *C. parvum* oocysts in soil was investigated in a series of batch equilibrium experiments. When combined with soil particles, and in presence of $CaCl_2$ solution, the oocysts were removed from the suspension with a high rate (**Table 4**). The results summarized in **Table 5** showed that oocysts, in the solution of NaBr, were transferred to the solid phase, suggesting a chemical environment favorable for the retention of oocysts. In addition the alkaline pH measured in the physicochemical

Samples	C_0 (oocysts)	C_e (oocyst/L)	V_{CaCl_2}	Msol(g)	q_e (oocyst.L/g)
Cc1	1ml contains 40.000	0	39	4	400
Cc2	2ml contains 80.000	0	38	4	800
Cc3	3ml contains 120.000	0	37	4	1200
Cc4	4ml contains 160.000	0	36	4	1600
Cc5	5ml contains 200.000	13	35	4	2000
Cc6	6ml contains 240.000	13	34	4	2400

Table 4.
Results of the test absorption studies between oocysts and soil with $CaCl_2$.

Sample	C0 (oocysts)	Ce (oocyst/L)	V_{NaBr}	Msol(g)	q_e (oocyst.L/g)
Cc1	1ml contains 40.000	0	39	4	400
Cc2	2ml contains 80.000	0	38	4	800
Cc3	3ml contains 120.000	0	37	4	1200
Cc4	4ml contains 160.000	0	36	4	1600
Cc5	5ml contains 200.000	0	35	4	2000
Cc6	6ml contains 240.000	0	34	4	2400

Table 5.
Results of the test absorption studies between oocysts and soil with NaBr.

analyses of the soil can increase the negative charge of zeta potential of oocysts and ultimately reduce the retention capacity of the soil. This could explain the presence of oocysts in groundwater. However, interactions between small colloid particles, the size of *C. parvum* oocysts, and small soil particles, typically the clay-sized fraction (<2 μm), depend to a large extent on electrostatic and other surface forces. Hence, surface charge, characterized as electrophoretic mobility or zeta potential, may govern the interaction between oocysts and soil particles [72]. Furthermore keeping the soil in its natural condition including clay particles and organic matter, which are important for adhesion and may be high in water suspensions in the environment. The association of oocysts with clay minerals has been attributed to high cation exchange capacity (CEC) of clays [72]. This could explain adsorption of oocysts on soil particles in the test batch. The high content of organic material obtained may affect the transport of pathogenic microorganisms in the soil to promote their retention [73]. Tufenkji et al. found that the oocyst removal efficiency depended on ionic strength and solution pH.

Other studies have reported that the ionic strength of the solution can influence the behavior of oocysts in the soil. Increasing the ionic strength of the water can alter the hydrophobic behavior of oocysts. According to the Debye-Hückel equation, the two solutions used for this study had different ionic strength. This distribution can be explained by the retention of oocysts in the solution containing $CaCl_2$ (**Table 4**). While for NaBr, for the same ionic strength, the activity of Na^+ ions is almost identical to the activity of Br^- ions. There is a total transfer of the oocysts of the aqueous phase to the solid phase (**Table 5**). Indeed, changes in particle surface chemistry can have a significant influence on particle aggregation and adhesion [62, 74]. An improved understanding of the influence of oocyst purification and handling methods on oocyst surface chemistry and subsequent stability (vide infra) in water may lead to more effective oocyst removal in engineered processes [75]. Thomas et al. [76] recently reported that oocysts suspended in $CaCl_2$ solutions had near-zero electrophoretic mobility. Brush et al. [62] have reported that variations in observed electrophoretic mobilities were caused by dissimilarities in purification techniques.

5.1 Dynamics of pollution of water resources in the city of Les Cayes

Pollution dynamics of water resources refer in this chapter to all mechanisms resulting from anthropogenic activities that contribute to the degradation of water quality. This dynamic is the result of a series of actions to be closely linked to spatial development, population growth, and especially to inaction of the public authorities.

The groundwater of the Plaine des Cayes is an important resource. From an ecological point of view, they represent a quantitatively large water reserve and contribute to the feeding of many lakes and rivers. In addition, they provide a significant part of the water supply for the population. The mode of supply is made from groundwater withdrawals with the installation of wells and boreholes and by capture of sources. Distribution takes place from networks, private connections, and public fountains. According to the data of the information, the water of the municipal system is fed by two boreholes with a flow of 66 l/s and an average production of the order of 10,134 m^3/day.

Work carried out on the groundwaters of the country indicates their saline contamination [77] and the presence of pathogenic microorganisms (S/Committee on drinking water and human waste disposal, 1991) [78] and chemical pollutants [79]. In Haiti, several factors include the lack of a system for the collection and drainage of urban effluents, the absence of wastewater treatment plants, the discharge of septic tank effluents into karstic and alluvial formations, as well as the construction of latrines in the aforementioned geological formations, contribute to microbiological contamination of groundwater. A total of 110 fecal coliforms per 100 ml of water was detected in the water distributed by the public service of the city of Les Cayes (S/Committee on drinking water and human waste disposal, 1991).

Based on findings, it appears that the population of the city of Les Cayes resorts to the use of nonreturn latrines and WC with septic tanks, improved latrines, and with non-defined systems (defecation in open air) for the evacuation of their excreta. In the same manner, the people of Les Cayes use various channels for the evacuation of their solid waste: direct removal by the trucks and other discharges into waterways, wastelands, drains, etc. Quite often, the waste which undergoes putrefaction on garbage heaps as well as it does in trash bins produces an extremely toxic liquid called lixiviant. This situation can contribute to the contamination of the water table's water resources through human fecal matter.

All of these pose serious threats to water resources that are heavily exploited in the area through wells, springs, and boreholes. Groundwater is generally polluted by the excreta. People are digging latrines until they reach the surface of the water table. After a rise of a water table above the ground surface, the excreta can be mobilized by the runoff and can be dispersed all over the surface and can pose a significant pollution hazard. It is clear that solid waste and wastewater have as receptacle the aquatic ecosystems and greatly contribute to altering the quality of water resources.

5.1.1 Health impact related to the degradation of water resources

Regarding cryptosporidiosis in Haiti, in the early 2000s, a series of environmental investigations had been conducted in Port-au-Prince and its surroundings, Les Cayes, and Cap-Haitien to identify human contamination sources. So far, these surveys consisted only in detecting *Cryptosporidium* oocysts in the environment by screening different types of water (surface water, groundwater, public water supplies) used by the population [10–12]. Cryptosporidiosis is one of the most frequent causes of diarrhea in Haiti. Transmission in young children, HIV-infected individuals, and people living in low socioeconomic conditions is probably due to consumption of water or food contaminated by *Cryptosporidium* oocysts. In tropical areas and under unfavorable socioeconomic conditions, cryptosporidiosis of the child is associated with a risk of prolonged diarrhea, malnutrition, and possibly psychomotor retardation and lectin-related mannose deficiency [80].Cryptosporidiosis is responsible for 17.5% of acute diarrhea cases in children <2 years old [81] and for 30% of HIV patients with chronic diarrhea [82]. Cryptosporidiosis is associated with Haitian children with malnutrition and lectin-related mannose deficiency. In a study conducted in Port-au-Prince, the presence of *Cryptosporidium* oocysts was shown in 158 people (a prevalence of 10.3%). Among these individuals, 56 out of 57 (98%) adults and 7 out of 36 (19%) children were HIV^{+}. Genotyping identified three species: 59% *C. hominis*, 38% *C. parvum*, and 3% *C. felis* [12]. It is one of the leading causes of morbidity and mortality in people with AIDS [82]. Cryptosporidiosis is considered as a significant health problem in Haiti where cryptosporidiosis appears to be closely related to environmental issues. Water and sanitation are environmental issues to their very core and together constitute one of the top drivers of development. Water and sanitation provision have an impact on the health of the environment, through downstream pollution in particular.

5.1.2 Environmental impacts related to the degradation of water resources

Pollution of water resources has a particular impact on the environment, especially since water is an essential component of the ecosystem. Water pollution affects air, soil, and plants. In this, the stagnation of wastewater in the open spaces generates foul odors which constitute an inconvenience for the population. This mode of management or disposal of wastewater causes inter alia disturbances in the nutrient cycle, changes in the structure and functioning of the biotic community, and a biological imbalance in aquatic ecosystems. The high pollutant loads contained in water surface are at the origin of eutrophication. In addition, the weakness of the collection system means that solid waste is dispersed in gullies in public squares, in public markets, and accumulates in open drainage channels contributing to the degradation of the environment. In addition, the accumulation of organic waste in the urban environment favors murine swarming, a reservoir of *Cryptosporidium muris*, a species recently found in humans in Peru [83]. Leachate from leachate is leaking into the drinking water system, with old and poorly maintained pipelines on the surface in many streets. These conditions of urban insalubrity explain the particularly high rate of contamination by *Cryptosporidium* oocysts of water for human consumption. The impact on the environment affects the attractiveness of the city of Les Cayes.

6. Conclusion

Pollution of water resources in developing countries is a public health problem. This problem affects everyday life and the living standards of urban populations. In the urban areas of poor countries, uncontrolled population growth puts severe pressure on existing natural resources, particularly water resources, resulting in accelerated environmental degradation. In particular, the water resources of the city of Les Cayes are subject to various pressures on a daily basis as a result of poor sanitation and poor solid waste management. To understand the dynamics of water resource pollution by microorganisms, a study on the behavior of *Cryptosporidium* oocysts under chemical conditions was carried out. The objective of this study was to investigate the behavior of *Cryptosporidium* oocysts under chemical conditions and soil characteristics in saturated porous media and to describe also the water pollution dynamics of *Cryptosporidium* oocysts. Batch equilibrium tests were used to describe the partitioning of *Cryptosporidium* particles between solid and liquid phases and play a significant role in the oocyst removal from the pore fluid. Therefore it is necessary to reduce the level of exposure of the population of Les Cayes through the construction of livestock farms to prevent the free movement of animals in the city, the elimination of wild dumps, and the treatment of urban effluents, latrine sludge, and septic tanks. It is important to regularly monitor water quality (monitoring) and evaluate progress. Good management of water resources on our study site requires close collaboration between research institutes, water companies, and health authorities.

Author details

Ketty Balthazard-Accou[1,2*], Evens Emmanuel[3], Patrice Agnamey[4,5] and Christian Raccurt[6]

1 Laboratoire de Qualité de l'Eau de l'Environnement, Université Quisqueya, Port-au-Prince, Haïti

2 Association Haïtienne Femmes, Science et Technologie, Port-au-Prince, Haïti

3 École doctorale "Société et Environnement", Université Quisqueya, Port-au-Prince, Haïti

4 Laboratoire de Parasitologie—Mycologie, Hôpital Sud, CHU d'Amiens

5 AGIR—Agents Infectieux, Résistance et Chimiothérapie, UFR de Pharmacie, Amiens, France

6 Faculté des Sciences de la Santé, Université Quisqueya, Port-au-Prince, Haïti

*Address all correspondence to: kettybal@gmail.com

References

[1] Eriksson E, Baun A, Mikkelsen PS, Ledin A. Risk assessment of xenobiotics in stormwater discharged to Harrestrup Å, Denmark. Desalination. 2007;**215**:187-197

[2] Zhang Q, Li ZW, Zeng GM, Li JB, Fang Y, Yuan QS, et al. Assessment of surface water quality using multivariate statistical techniques in red soil hilly region: A case study of Xiangjiang watershed, China. Environmental Monitoring and Assessment. 2009;**152**:123-131

[3] Fifi U. Impacts des eaux pluviales urbaines sur les eaux souterraines dans les pays en développement—mécanismes de transfert des métaux lourds à travers un sol modèle de Port-au-Prince, Haïti [Thèse de Doctorat]. Lyon: INSA de Lyon; 2010. p. 260

[4] Ghosh AR, Qureshi MS, Kim JI, Zalduendo J. Surges. Journal of International Economics. 2014;**92**(2):266-285

[5] Krishnan RS, Srinivasan R, Devanarayanan S. Thermal Expansion of Crystals: International Series in the Science of the Solid State (Vol. 22). Elsevier; 2013

[6] Maillard P, Santos NAP. A spatial-statistical approach for modeling the effect of non-point source pollution on different water quality parameters in the Velhas river watershed-Brazil. Journal of Environmental Management. 2008;**86**(1):158-170

[7] Rashid Abo ul HM, Malik MM, Mukhtar S. Urbanization and its effects on water resources: An exploratory analysis. Asian Journal of Water, Environment and Pollution. 2018;**15**(1):67-74. DOI: 10.3233/AJW-180007

[8] Emmanuel E. Evaluation des risques sanitaires et écotoxicologiques liés aux effluents hospitaliers [Thèse de Doctorat]. Lyon: INSA de Lyon; 2004. p. 257

[9] Pitt R, Clark S, Field R. Groundwater contamination potential from stormwater infiltration practices. Urban Water. 1999;**1**:217-236

[10] Balthazard-Accou K, Emmanuel E, Agnamey P, Brasseur P, Totet A, Raccurt CP. *Cryptosporidium* oocysts transmission in the aquatic environment of Haiti. In: Laboy-Nieves EN, Goosen MFA, Emmanuel E, editors. Environmental and Human Health. CRC Press/Taylor & Francis Group; 2010. pp. 201-214

[11] Brasseur P, Eyma E, Li X, Verdier Ri, Agnamey P, Liautaud B, et al. Circulation des oocystes de Cryptosporidium dans les eaux de surface et de distribution par adduction publique à Port-au-Prince, Haïti. In: Colloque International Gestion Intégrée de l'Eau en Haïti, Actes du Colloque; 2002. pp. 172-175

[12] Raccurt CP, Brasseur P, Verdier RI, Li X, Eyma E, Panier Stockman C, et al. Cryptosporidiose humaine et espèces en cause en Haïti. Tropical Medicine and International Health. 2006;**11**:929-934

[13] Damiani C, Balthazard-Accou K, Clervil E, Diallo A, Da Costa C, Emmanuel E, et al. Cryptosporidiosis in Haiti: Surprisingly low level of species diversity revealed by molecular characterization of *Cryptosporidium* oocysts from surface water and groundwater. Parasite. 2013;**20**:45. Available from: www.parasite-journal.org

[14] Balthazard-Accou K, Emmanuel E, Agnamey P, Brasseur P, Lilite O, Totet A, et al. Presence of *Cryptosporidium* oocysts and Giardia Cysts in the surface water and groundwater in the City of Cayes, Haití. Aqua-LAC. 2009;**1**:63-71

[15] Balthazard-Accou K. Contamination microbiologique des eauxsouterraines de la ville des Cayes, Haïti. Evaluation des risques pour la santédes consommateurs [Thèse de Doctorat]. Amiens: Université de Picardie Jules Verne; 2011. p. 208

[16] Balthazard-Accou K, Fif U, Agnamey P, Casimir JA, Brasseur P, Emmanuel E. Influence of ionic strength and soil characteristics on the behavior of *Cryptosporidium* oocysts in saturated porous media. Chemosphere. 2014;**103**:114-120

[17] Clode PL, Koh WH, Thompson RC. Life without a host cell: What is *Cryptosporidium*? Trends in Parasitology. 2015;**31**:614-624

[18] Armon R, Gold D, Zuckerman U, Eyal Kurzbaum E. Environmental aspect of cryptosporidium. Journal of Veterinary Medicine and Research. 2016;**3**(2):1048

[19] Bonnard R. Le risque biologique et la méthode d'évaluation du risque. Paris: Institut National de l'Environnement Industriel et des Risques; 2001. p. 70. INERIS (DRC-01-25419-ERSA-RBn-383)

[20] Carey CM, Lee H, Trevors JT. Biology, persistence and detection of *Cryptosporidium parvum* and *Cryptosporidium hominis* oocyst. Water Research. 2004;**38**:818-862

[21] Robertson LJ, Campbell AT, Smith HV. Survival of *Cryptosporidium parvum* oocysts under various environmental pressures. Applied and Environmental Microbiology. 1992;**58**:3494-3500

[22] Jenkins MB, Bowman DD, Fogarty EA, Ghiiorse WC. *Cryptosporidium parvum* oocyst inactivation in three soil types at various temperatures and water potentials. Soil Biology and Biochemistry. 2002;**34**:1101-1109

[23] Fayer R, Trout JM, Jenkins MC. Infectivity of *Cryptosporidium parvum* oocysts stored in water at environmental temperatures. Journal of Parasitology. 1998;**84**:1165-1169

[24] Fayer R, Trout JM, Nerad T. Effects of a wide range of temperatures on infectivity of *Cryptosporidium parvum* oocysts. The Journal of Eukaryotic Microbiology. 1996;**43**:64S

[25] Chauret C, Armstrong N, Fisher J, Sharma R, Springthorpe S, Sattar S. Correlating *Cryptosporidium* and Giardia with microbial indicators. Journal of the American Water Works Association. 1995;**87**:76-84

[26] Liu W, An W, Jeppesen E, Ma J, Min Y, Dennis T. Modelling the fate and transport of Cryptosporidium, a zoonotic and waterborne pathogen, in the Daning River watershed of the three Gorges Reservoir Region, China. Journal of Environmental Management;**232**:462-474. DOI: 10.1016/j.jenvman.2018.10.064

[27] Liu J, Platts-Mills JA, Juma J, Kabir F, Nkeze J, Okoi C, et al. Use of quantitative molecular diagnostic methods to identify causes of diarrhoea in children: A reanalysis of the GEMS case-control study. Lancet. 2016;**388**:1291-1301. DOI: 10.1016/S0140-6736(16)31529-X

[28] Gatei W, Wamae CN, Mbae C, Waruru A, Mulinge E, Waithera T, et al. Cryptosporidiosis: Prevalence, genotype analysis, and symptoms associated with infections in children in Kenya. The American Journal of Tropical Medicine and Hygiene. 2006;**75**(1):78-82

[29] Craun GF, Calderon RL. Observational epidemiologic studies of endemic waterborne risks: Cohort, case-control, time-series, and ecologic studies. Journal of Water and Health. 2006;**4**:101-119

[30] Xiao L, Cama VA. Cryptosporidium and Cryptosporidiosis Foodborne Parasites. Berlin, Germany:

Springer; 2018. pp. 73-117. DOI: 10.1007/978-3-319-67664-7-5

[31] Kato S, Jenkins M, Fogarty E, Bowman D. *Cryptosporidium parvum* oocyst inactivation in field soil and its relation to soil characteristics: Analyses using the geographic information systems. Science of the Total Environment. 2004;**321**(1-3):47-58. DOI: 10.1016/j.scitotenv.2003.08.027

[32] Chappell CL, Okhuysen PC, Sterling CR, Wang C, Jakubowski W, Dupont HL. Infectivity of *Cryptosporidium parvum* in healthy adults with pre-existing anti-*Cryptosporidium parvum* serum immunoglobulin G. The American Journal of Tropical Medicine and Hygiene. 1999;**60**(1):157-164. DOI: 10.4269/ajtmh.1999.60.157

[33] Mac Kenzie WR, Hoxie NJ, Proctor ME, Gradus MS, Blair KA, Peterson DE, et al. A massive outbreak in Milwaukee of *Cryptosporidium* infection transmitted through the public water supply. The New England Journal of Medicine. 1994;**331**(3):161-167

[34] Robertson LJ, Chalmers RM. Foodborne cryptosporidiosis: Is there really more in Nordic countries? Trends in Parasitology. 2013;**29**(1):3-9

[35] Utaaker KS, Skjerve E, Robertson LJ. Keeping it cool: Survival of Giardia cysts and *Cryptosporidium* oocysts on lettuce leaves. International Journal of Food Microbiology. 2017;**255**:51-57

[36] Åberg R, Sjöman M, Hemminki K, Pirnes A, Räsänen S, Kalanti A, et al. *Cryptosporidium parvum* caused a large outbreak linked to frisée salad in Finland, 2012. Zoonoses and Public Health. 2015;**62**(8):618-624

[37] McKerr C, Adak GK, Nichols G, Gorton R, Chalmers RM, Kafatos G, et al. An outbreak of *Cryptosporidium parvum* across England & Scotland associated with consumption of fresh pre-cut salad leaves, May 2012. PLoS ONE. 2012;**10**(5):e0125955

[38] Cook N, Lim YAL. Giardia duodenalis: Part 1: Contamination of fresh produce. In: Robertson LJ, Smith H, editors. Foodborne Protozoan Parasites. Hauppauge: Nova Publishers; 2012. pp. 105-107

[39] Atwill ER, Hou L, Karle BM, Harter T, Tate KW, Dahlgren RA. Transport of *Cryptosporidium parvum* oocysts through vegetated buffer strips and estimated filtration efficiency. Applied and Environmental Microbiology. 2002;**68**:5517-5527

[40] Davies CM, Ferguson CM, Kaucner C, Krogh M, Altavilla N, Deere DA, et al. Dispersion and transport of *Cryptosporidium* oocysts from fecal pats under simulated rainfall events. Applied and Environmental Microbiology. 2004;**70**:1151-1159

[41] Bradford SA, Bettahar M. Straining attachment and detachment of *Cryptosporidium* oocysts in saturated porous media. Journal of Environmental Quality. 2005;**34**:469-478

[42] Tufenkji N, Dixon DR, Considine R, Drummond CJ. Multi-scale *Cryptosporidium*/sand interactions in water treatment. Water Research. 2006;**40**:3315-3331

[43] Byrd TL, Walz JY. Investigation of the interaction force between *Cryptosporidium parvum* oocysts and solid surfaces. Langmuir. 2007;**23**:7475-7483

[44] Liu Y, Janjaroen D, Kuhlenschmidt MS, Kuhlenschmidt TB, Nguyen TH. Deposition of *Cryptosporidium parvum* oocysts on natural organic matter surfaces: Microscopic evidence for secondary minimum deposition in a radial stagnation point flow cell. Langmuir. 2009;**3**:1594-1605

[45] Janjaroen D, Liu Y, Kuhlenschmidt MS, Kuhlenschmidt TB, Nguyen TH. Role of divalent cations on deposition of *Cryptosporidium parvum* oocysts on natural organic matter surfaces. Environmental Science & Technology. 2010;**44**:4519-4524

[46] Petersen HH, Enemark HL, Olsen A, Mostofa Amin MG, Dalsgaarda A. Transport of *Cryptosporidium parvum* oocysts in soil columns following applications of raw and separated liquid slurries. Applied and Environmental Microbiology. 2012;**78**:5994-6000

[47] McLaughlin SJ, Kalita PK, Kuhlenschmidt MS. Fate of *Cryptosporidium parvum* oocysts within soil, water, and plant environment. Journal of Environmental Management. 2013;**131**:121-128

[48] Darnault CJG, Peng Z, Yu C, Li B, Jacobson AR, Baveye PC. Movement of *Cryptosporidium parvum* oocysts through soils without preferential pathways: Exploratory test. Frontiers in Environmental Science. 2017;**5**:39. DOI: 10.3389/fenvs.2017.00039

[49] Current W. Cryptosporidium: Its biology and potential for environmental transmission. CRC Critical Reviews in Environmental Control. 1987;**17**:21-51

[50] Kuznar Z, Elimelech M. *Cryptosporidium* oocysts surface macromolecules significantly hinder oocyst attachment. Environmental Science and Technology. 2006;**40**:1837-1842

[51] Considine RF, Dixon DR, Drummond CJ. Laterally-resolved force microscopy of biological microspheres-oocysts of *Cryptosporidium parvum*. Langmuir. 2000;**16**:1323-1330

[52] Considine RF, Dixon DR, Drummond CJ. Oocysts of *Cryptosporidium parvum* and model sand surfaces in aqueous solutions: An atomic force microscope (AFM) study. Water Research. 2002;**36**:3421-3428

[53] Drozd C, Schwartzbrod J. Hydrophobic and electrostatic cell surface properties of *Cryptosporidium parvum*. Apply and Environmental Microbiology. 1996;**62**:1227-1232

[54] Hsu BM, Huang CP. Influence of ionic strength and pH on hydrophobicity and zeta potential of Giardia and *Cryptosporidium*. Colloids and Surfaces A: Physicochemical and Engineering Aspects. 2002;**3**:201-206

[55] Karaman ME, Pashley RM, Bustamante H, Shanker SR. Microelectrophoresis of *Cryptosporidium parvum* oocysts in aqueous solutions of inorganic and surfactant cations. Colloids and Surfaces A: Physicochemical and Engineering Aspects. 1999;**146**:217-225

[56] Ongerth JE, Pecoraro JP. Electrophoretic mobility of *Cryptosporidium* oocysts and *Giardia* cysts. Journal of Environmental Engineering. 1996;**122**:228-231

[57] Thomas F, Bard E, Rouiller MC, Prelot B, Mathieu L. Filtration-elution of *Cryptosporidium* oocysts assisted by electrostatic interactions. Colloids and Surfaces A: Physicochemical and Engineering Aspects. 2001;**195**:135-142

[58] Searcy KE, Packman AI, Atwill ER, Harter T. Association of *Cryptosporidium parvum* with suspended particles: Impact on oocyst sedimentation. Applied and Environmental Microbiology. 2005;**71**:1072-1078

[59] Dai X, Boll J, Hayes ME, Aston DE. Adhesion of *Cryptosporidium parvum* and *Giardia lamblia* to solid surfaces: The role of surface charge and hydrophobicity. Colloids and Surfaces. B, Biointerfaces. 2004;**34**:259-263

[60] Kuznar ZA, Elimelech M. Adhesion kinetics of viable *Cryptosporidium parvum* oocysts to quartz surfaces.

Environmental Science & Technology. 2004;**38**:6839-6845

[61] Deyac KECV, López LMT, Agosto MG, Emmanuel E. The physical properties of *Cryptosporidium* oocysts and their adsorption to solid surfaces: A review. 2011

[62] Brush C, Walter M, Anguish L, Ghiorse W. Influence of pretreatment and experimental conditions on electrophoretic mobility and hydrophobicity of *Cryptosporidium parvum* oocyst. Applied an Environmental Microbiology. 1998;**64**(11):4439-4445

[63] Harvey RW, Garabedian SP. Use of colloid filtration theory in modeling movement of bacteria through a contaminated sandy aquifer. Environmental Science and Technology. 1991;**25**:178-185

[64] DeMarsily G. Quantitative Hydrogeology. 1st ed. San Diego, CA: Academic Press; 1986. 440p

[65] Ryan JN, Elimelech M. Colloid mobilization and transport in groundwater. Colloids and Surfaces A: Physicochemical and Engineering Aspects. 1996;**107**:1-56

[66] Logan BE, Jewett DG, Arnold RG, Bouwer EJ, O'Melia CR. Clarification of clean-bed filtration models. Journal of Environmental Engineering. 1995;**121**(12):869-873

[67] Rajagopalan R, Tien C. Trajectory analysis of deep-bed filtration with the sphere-in-cell porous media model. AICHE Journal. 1976;**22**(3):523-533

[68] PNUD, Programme des Nations Unies pour le Développement. Développement et gestion des ressources en eau. In: Haïti: Disponibilité en eau et adéquation aux besoins. Volume VI Région Sud-Ouest. New-York (NY): PNUD; 1991. 70p

[69] Ministère de la Santé Publique. Analyse de la Situation Sanitaire (Haïti). Port-au-Prince: Imprimerie Henri Deschamps; 1998. 250p

[70] AFNOR NFT90-455. Qualité de l'eau. In: Recherche et Dénombrement D'oocystes de Cryptosporidium et de Kystes de Giardia—Méthode de Concentration et de Dénombrement. Association Française de Normalisation; 2001. 25p

[71] Hillel D. Environmental Soil Physics: Fundamentals, Applications and Environmental Considerations. Academic Press; 1998. 771p

[72] Peng X, Macdonald S, Murphy TM, Holden NM. The fate and transport of Cryptosporidium parvum oocysts in the soil. In: Ozkaraova Gungor BE, editor. Principles, Application and Assessment in Soil Science. Rijeka: InTech; 2011. pp. 179-192. ISBN: 978-953-307-740-6. Available from: http://www.intechopen.com/books/principlesapplication-and-assessment-in-soil-science/the-fate-and-transportof-cryptosporidium-parvum-oocysts-inthesoil

[73] Tufenkji N, Elimelech M. Spatial distributions of *Cryptosporidium* oocysts in porous media: Evidence for dual mode deposition. Environmental Science & Technology. 2005;**39**:3620-3629. DOI: 10.1021/es048289y

[74] Butkus MA, Grasso D. The impact of phosphate sorption on water treatment residual surface characteristics: Prelude to reuse. Environmental Engineering Science. 1999;**16**:117-129. DOI: 10.1089/ees.1999.16.117

[75] Butkus M, Bays J, Labare M. Influence of surface characteristics on the stability of *Cryptosporidium parvum* oocyst. Applied and Environmental Microbiology. 2003;**69**(7):3819-3825

[76] Thomas F, Bard E, Rouillier MC, Prelot B, Mathieu L. Filtration-elution

of *Cryptosporidium* oocysts assisted by electrostatic inter-actions. Colloids and Surfaces A: Physicochemical and Engineering Aspects. 2001;**195**:135-142

[77] Simonot M. Les Ressources en eau Souterraine de la région de Port-au-Prince. Situation Actuelle et Recommandation. Port-au-Prince: PNUD (Programme des Nations Unies pour le Développement; 1982. 52p

[78] Emmanuel E, Lindskog P. Regards sur la situation actuelle des ressources en eau de la République d'Haïti. In: Emmanuel E, Vermande P, editors. Actes du Colloque International Gestion Intégrée de l'Eau en Haïti. Port-au-Prince: Laboratoire de Qualité de l'Eau et de l'Environnement, Université Quisqueya; 2002. pp. 30-52

[79] Emmanuel E, Angerville R, Joseph O, Perrodin Y. Human health risk assessment of lead in drinking water: A case study from Port-au-Prince Haiti. International Journal of Environment and Pollution. 2007;**31**(3/4):280-291

[80] Kirrkpatrick BD, Danniels MM, Jean SS, Pape JW, Karp C, Litterger B, et al. *Cryptosporidiosis* stimulates an inflammatory intestinal response in malnourished Haitian children. Journal of Infectious Diseases. 2002;**186**:94-101

[81] Pape JW, Levine E, Beaulieu ME, Marshall F, Verdier R, Johnson WD Jr. Cryptosporidiosis in Haitian children. American Journal of Tropical Medicine and Hygiene. 1987;**36**:333-337

[82] Pape JW, Liautaud B, Thomas F, et al. The acquired immunodeficiency syndrome in Haiti. Annals of Internal Medicine. 1983;**103**:674-678

[83] Palmer CJ, Xiao L, Terashima A, et al. *Cryptosporidium muris*, a rodent pathogen, recovered from a human in Peru. Emerging Infectious Diseases. 2003;**9**:1174-1176

Chapter 3

Rainwater Harvesting Infrastructure Management

Mirzi Betasolo and Carl Smith

Abstract

As climate change impact is affecting all countries, water scarcity is continually a pressing issue to all countries in the world. The groundwater availability around the globe and locally such as in the ground of Papua New Guinea, Lae City, the garden city of the country, is also affected by the phenomenon. An alternative source such as the rainwater which across the globe is not equally shared thus harvesting it by creating an infrastructure for wider use needs management for sustainability. The study focuses on the management of a rainwater harvesting infrastructure (RHI) from its initial stage or conceptualization by designing using axiomatic design process and creating a model prototype to show the features of the infrastructure. The axiomatic design process in the design of the rainwater harvesting infrastructure shows the customer needs and functionality of the infrastructure for cost-wise management. The chapter provides information for a broader and more significant impact of providing and designing infrastructure for massive use.

Keywords: rainwater harvesting, infrastructure management, natural resource, a renewable resource, climate change, sustainability

1. Introduction to rainwater harvesting

This chapter discusses the rainwater harvesting infrastructure (RHI) management. Similar to any harvesting strategy such as in the farm, infrastructure is important to keep your harvest sustainable until the next harvest. Rainwater, like any other renewable resource, needs to be sustainable because, with human activities, the regular hydrologic cycle is affected by climate change (**Figure 1**). There are five processes at work in the hydrologic cycle: condensation, precipitation, inflitration, runoff, and evatranspiration [1]. These occur simultaneously and, result in precipitation when the conditions are suitable. Precipitation is a product of condensation of atmospheric water vapor and fall under gravity to the land surface as rain and infiltrates the soil or flows to the ocean as runoff, or surface water (e.g., lakes, streams, oceans, etc.), evaporates, returning moisture to the atmosphere, while vegetation returns water to the atmosphere by transpiration and the cycle continuous. For more understanding, necessary information on rainwater harvesting is discussed below.

1.1 What is rainwater harvesting?

Rainwater harvesting [2] is the capturing of rain from rooftops, catchments, local streams, seasonal floodwaters, and watershed management to conserve water; to provide drinking water, irrigation water, and groundwater recharge; and to

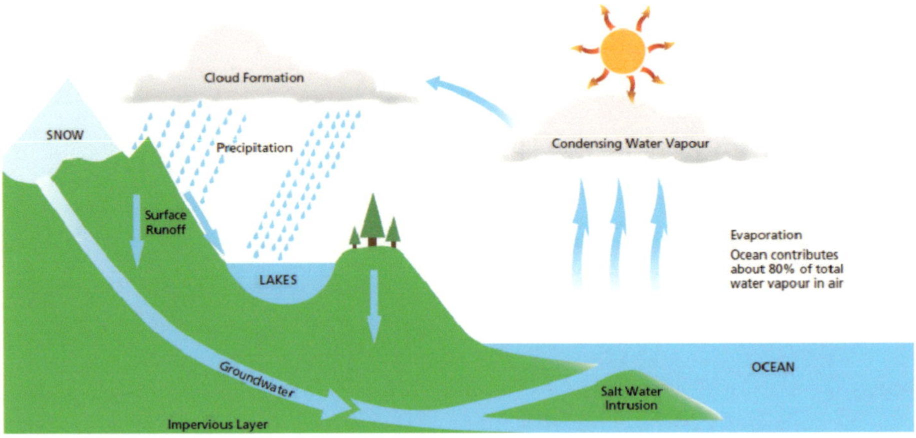

Figure 1.
Hydrologic cycle. (Adapted from NASA.)

reduce stormwater discharges, urban flood, water overloading in sewage treatment plants, and seawater ingress in coastal areas. It is an activity of direct or indirect collection of rainwater (**Table 1**).

The rainwater harvesting is a promising alternative infrastructure in the imminence of increasing water scarcity and escalating demand for water supply [3]. It maximizes water efficiency by capturing it rather than letting it run off. By doing so, it minimizes the increase in environmental impact from a large project in which the pressure on water supplies occurs. Allowing the rain to fall anywhere also allow deteriorating water quality and constrain the ability to meet the demand for fresh water from traditional sources as it goes to the drainage system instead of utilizing it for multiple functions. Therefore, rainwater harvesting augments availability of water, self-reliance, and sustainability.

1.2 What is a rainwater harvesting system?

For better understanding of the term rainwater harvesting system, we will define it here as a technology used to collect; convey rain for future use from relatively clean surfaces such as a roof, land surface, or rock catchment; and store it [4]. There are two classified practices in collecting rainwater from rainfall events. The two broad categories are land-based and roof-based. Land-based rainwater harvesting when runoff comes from land surfaces is collected in furrow dikes, ponds, tanks, and reservoirs. Roof-based rainwater harvesting comes from collecting rainwater runoff through roof surfaces which usually provides a much cleaner source of water for drinking purposes [5].

Due to the impact on climate change, a need for sustainable rainwater harvesting is a necessity. Thus, a sustainable rainwater harvesting system (SRHS) had been studied and is defined as the collection and storage of rainwater for human use in a manner that preserves and protects the environment and for the preservation of the natural resource (rainwater) for continuous supply today and in the future [6].

1.3 What is the rainwater harvesting infrastructure?

Rainwater harvesting was well defined above as collection and storage of rainwater for sustainability. Infrastructure is a fundamental physical and organizational structure and facilities that provide services to communities with high-cost

DOI: http://dx.doi.org/10.5772/intechopen.90342

Type of tests		Locations of sample tested						
		Erap	Boystown (Erap)	40 Mile	Balob T/C	Ampo	Martin Luther Seminary	WHO recommended
Test parameter	BOD	3.95 mg/L	3.95 mg/L	4.30 mg/L	3.8 mg/L	3.8 mg/L	3.1 mg/L	1 mg/L
	Hardness ($CaCO_3$)	250.5 mg/L	180.5 mg/L	238 mg/L	180 mg/L	214 mg/L	187 mg/L	100–500 mg/L
	Turbidity	3.54 NTU	13.13 NTU	2.0 NTU	0.21 NTU	0.27 NTU	0.21 NTU	1 NTU
	Calcium	25 mg/L	75 mg/L	63 mg/L	57 mg/L	68 mg/L	61 mg/L	75–200 mg/L
	Magnesium	4.55 mg/L	20 mg/L	47 mg/L	8.9 mg/L	11 mg/L	8.6 mg/L	30–150 mg/L

Table 1.
Table of pollution of groundwater taken from wells in Lae City.

investments or capital equipment such as the communal rainwater harvesting that are vital to the country's economic development and prosperity. The infrastructure is essential for any faster economic growth and alleviation of poverty in the country. The presence of an infrastructure (such as water supply, sewerage, roads, public space, electricity, bridges, tunnels, railways, canals, dams, building, airports, etc.) helps in increasing the overall productivity of the country's economy. In this chapter, the infrastructure is rainwater harvesting infrastructure.

The image shows an example of a rainwater harvesting infrastructure in Elisabeth, Jamaica (one of the author's home country, as shown in **Figure 2**). This method of harvesting rainwater is through a public infrastructure that can cater to the growing population of the city.

1.4 Rainwater harvesting technologies

For an understanding of this section, technologies used in rainwater harvesting are discussed here. There are several rainwater harvesting technologies such as rooftop, in situ, surface water, and groundwater recharge.

1.4.1 Rooftop

Rooftop rainwater harvesting technologies, according to the UNFCCC, are rainwater harvesting system that is a simple technology that promotes sustainable rainwater management and uses the roof as a catchment. The system comprises of three (3) basic elements such as catchment area (represented by the roof), conveyance system (gutters), and storage (tank). An example of a rooftop rainwater harvesting system is shown in **Figure 3**.

1.4.2 In situ

The in situ technology is a method where the storage of collected rainwater in a direct way is utilized immediately. For example, in arid and semiarid regions, the storage for the maximum amount of rainwater during the wet season is made for use at a later time when rain is low during the dry season, especially for agricultural

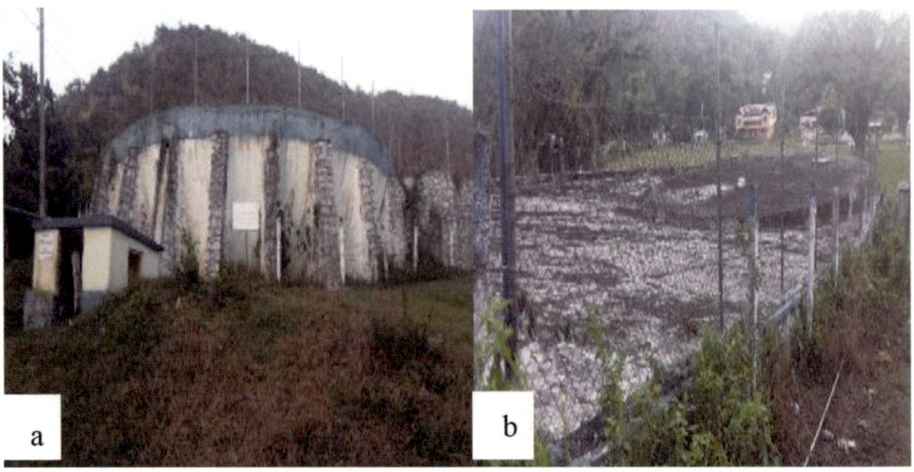

Figure 2.
(a) An elevated rainwater concrete catchment of Elisabeth, Jamaica; (b) the surface runoff and the storage tank of Elisabeth, Jamaica RHI. (Adapted from Betasolo and Smith, 2017.)

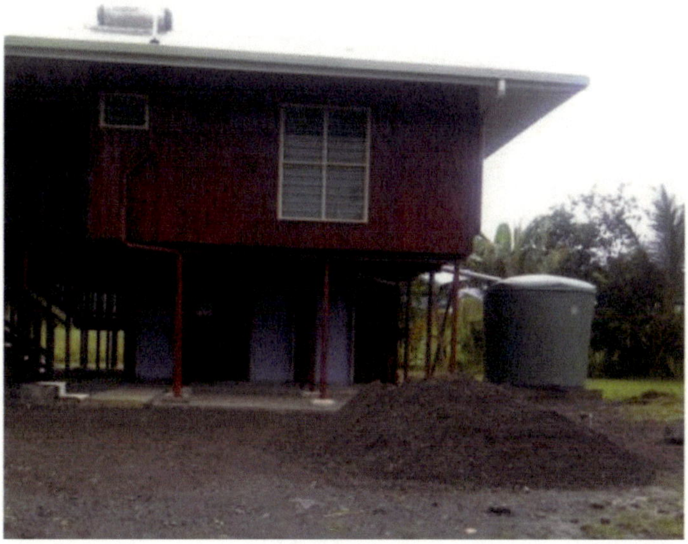

Figure 3.
Rainwater harvesting system (RWHS) via rooftop at Papua New Guinea University of Technology. (Adapted from Betasolo and Smith, 2017.)

and domestic water supply. This technique as other rainfall harvesting systems has three components: a collection, a conveyance system, and a storage area.

An example of in situ rainwater harvesting used in the arid and semiarid regions of Northeastern Brazil and Paraguay is primarily for irrigation purposes. The rainwater harvesting in situ in Brazil includes site preparation of agricultural areas which uses Topographic Depressions as Rainfall Harvesting Areas. *Tajamares* are constructed in areas of low topography used for rainwater storage with clay soils at least 3 m deep that served as distribution canals that convey water from the storage area to the areas of use which is the practice in Paraguay [5].

1.4.3 Surface water

Surface water is water on the surface found on wetlands that is nonsaline and is replenished by one of the processes in the hydrologic cycle—precipitation. The surface water supports the replenishment of groundwater aquifer supply if it is channeled efficiently. In most urban areas, the surface water is wasted and polluted. The wasting can be mitigated with proper utilization of surface water from rain via rainwater harvesting and storing it into the aquifer. An example is shown in **Figure 4**.

1.4.4 Groundwater recharge

Groundwater recharge is a process where groundwater is supported by several techniques to add or bring back the health of the groundwater for sustainability. It can be upstream or downstream discharge such as areas close to mountain peaks because the precipitation is higher than in the adjacent lowlands. The shallow groundwater discharges directly to the valleys, and too low-lying zones and the deep groundwater discharge directly to the oceans through return flow on irrigation, leakage from runoff, and wastewater collection system [6, 7].

The pollution of groundwater is inevitable by an impairment of water quality by chemicals, heat, or bacteria that may not necessarily create public health hazards

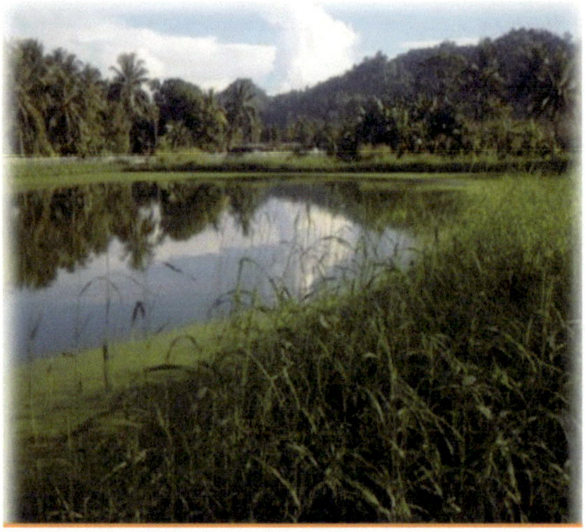

Figure 4.
Surface water found in Papua New Guinea University of Technology.

but does adversely affect the quality of water for domestic, farm, municipal, or industrial use [8]. The human body of an average adult contains up to 55-60% water [9]. Therefore people's health is dependent on a clean supply of water and safe sanitation. It is estimated that 50% of the people living in developing countries are suffering from water-related diseases caused directly by infection or indirectly by disease-carrying organisms that breed in water, such as mosquitoes causing malaria, diarrhea, infections by parasites, and river blindness that are among the most widespread diseases. Study of Betasolo et al. is an example of groundwater pollution where BOD and turbidity level exceeds the standard. The study area is the industrial hub of Papua New Guinea (PNG), and for the most urbanized country, the pollution is much higher than that of PNG. The tabulated data comes from the result of a test in a National Analytical and Testing Service Laboratory (NATSL) of the Papua New Guinea University of Technology, and the result is compared to the World Health Organization (WHO) standards.

1.4.5 Fog and dew

The highlands of Papua New Guinea experience for (cloud that is at the ground) as temperature ranges from 18 to 23°C such that the dew can be collected (became tiny droplets of water) similar to rainwater harvesting for drinking. An example of such method is the one used by a Canadian nonprofit organization supporting safe drinking water at the region such as FogQuest who collect fog at 0.05 to 0.5 g of water from an instrument that looks like tall volleyball nets (made of polypropylene or polyethylene mesh) hanged to capture the water droplets [10].

Other regions (desert) similar to PNG may have the opportunity to collect rainwater produced from fog during winter period. I have lived sometime in those regions and experienced the dampness of some items left outside (balcony).

2. Importance of rainwater harvesting infrastructure

Rainwater is a resource as a result of the hydrologic cycle. Humans need water for various uses such as drinking water and save high-quality drinking water sources. It is used as utility water (i.e., flushing) to reduce the potable water consumption and minimize the volume of generated wastewater that can be utilized for irrigation water and groundwater recharge or replenishing groundwater levels. Rainwater harvesting will relieve the pressure on sewers, and it reduces stormwater discharges and water overloading in sewage treatment plants. It acts as an environmental measure to mitigate floods by reducing urban flood and reduce seawater ingress, sediment transport, or soil erosions to coastal areas.

2.1 Water scarcity

Water supply scarcity is a pressing issue as population demand is increasing geometrically. In the overall earth's water supply, fresh water amounts only to 0.62%, and the amount of fresh water in the globe are decreasing as affected by climate change in its natural availability in lakes, rivers, and groundwater [11, 12]. A Ceres study [13] reported that water scarcity attributes to the following conditions: inadequate natural resources (physical water scarcity) and poor management of the sufficient available water resources (economic water scarcity).

For global identification of water scarcity, the reader can participate in an interactive map available in https://waterscarcityatlas.org/. A scenario on water scarcity can be derived and produced a map for the country's water scarcity condition. As of 2006 records PNG water scarcity status is "of no scarcity", but reports show that the sustainable access to improved drinking water and improved sanitation is still 45% (40–45%) which falls below the threshold to support the increasing populations of Papua New Guinea [14, 15]. Such population will be needing more access to water of which the PNG government's goal to provide by 2030 at least a 70% access to water is critiqued by the World Bank that they are not even on track to meet either the millennium goal or its national development targets [15]. The average monthly precipitation in mm is 260.37 summarized from 30-year records (1900–2012) of the World Bank on PNG's monthly average as it is an ideal measurement to assess climate patterns studied over a long time [16, 17].

2.2 Rainwater availability

Rainwater availability needs to be checked in assessing the feasibility of developing an infrastructure. To determine the factor to whether rainwater harvesting (RWH) is a viable water supply system is the rainfall pattern over the year. Tropical climate with short (1–4 months) dry seasons and multiple high-intensity rainstorms like in Lae City known for its name as Rainy Lae of Papua New Guinea is a most suitable condition for water harvesting. Also, rainwater harvesting is most valuable in wet tropical climates like PNG, where the water quantity of surface water varies and passes the general rule for precipitation of over 50 mm/month. Thus the discussion in most scenario used is of Papua New Guinea (PNG), a tropical country.

PNG has annual average rainfall is 3142 mm [19], an ideal water harvesting capability. However, the condition of most of the population have limited access to water supply. No access to water supply in settlement area as the water provider is unable to service them due to customary land issue. Ninety percent of the country's land is customary land which due to many ownership hinder the development of the property. Few others who can afford to dig and buy a pump have access to groundwater [18]. Other use the rooftop to harvest rainwater since Lae City has a rainfall that ranges from 4000 to 5800 annually [17].

However, the current strategies of rooftop rainwater harvesting on access to sustainable water and sanitation cannot keep pace with rapid population growth that needs to be addressed to meet the MDG targets. Unless an RWH system infrastructure portfolio of significant investment is provided that can meet the increasing population demand to sustainable water supply and sanitation, the national goals to 2030 are also unlikely to be achieved. Therefore, proper management of rainwater resource for sustainability by creating an infrastructure is the aim of this chapter to mitigate the impact of water scarcity while there is an available untapped resource.

3. Types of rainwater harvesting

To further understand why rainwater harvesting infrastructure is important to sustain an increasing population, a discussion of the types of rainwater harvesting is presented in this section.

3.1 Rainwater harvesting via the roof

Rainwater harvesting via roof had been the source for domestic water supply in Papua New Guinea according to study of Betasolo et al. [17] by harvesting water through roof and collecting the rainwater with Tuffa tank [8] as shown in **Figure 3**. The roof is a collection area and the first contact to collect the rainwater. How effective and efficient the collection depends on the material of the roof, how the roof is build, and the quality of rainwater. From the roof, the rainwater is conveyed through gutters or conveyors or pipes for storage. The roof materials consists of inert material such as galvanized, wood, aluminum, plastic, glass, and fiberglass to maintain good quality of rainwater harvest.

The rainwater storage connecting the roof is made from an inert material such as corrugated galvanized iron, plastic, reinforced concrete, stainless steel, and fiberglass constructed as a separate unit from the building but connected via pipe systems.

3.2 Rainwater harvesting via catchments

The harvesting of rainwater is played by the catchments. A catchment is a collection of rainfall through a natural drainage area or natural landscape. A catchment area is a geographical area in which the river and its tributaries are drained or funneled. Papua New Guinea has large local streams (basins) such as Sepik River (the largest catchment of 78,000 km^2), Fly River (61,000 km^2), Purari River (33,670 km^2), Markham River (12,000 km^2), and Busu River. Markham River and Busu River are located closely to Lae City.

3.3 Rainwater harvesting via local streams seasonal floodwaters

Rainwater harvesting through local streams from floodwaters is harvesting rainwater that fall into the local streams, increasing the capacity of the streams and become floodwater affecting many of the vegetation. On the other hand, harvesting floodwater can support the needs of water on land irrigation as there are no irrigation facilities available in the country but rainfall to support the subsistence farming of most of the population. Rainwater harvesting through local streams also will provide groundwater recharge and decrease of salt water ingress on areas near the coastal line such as Lae City of Papua New Guinea that rely solely on groundwater as a water supply in the urban area.

3.4 Rainwater harvesting via watershed management to conserve water

Watershed development and management is a technique to conserve water. However, it does not directly provide the water supply of the people, but it supports a continuous supply of the resource. Thus, management of the watershed, which also involved a great sum of the fund, is as equally important as creating the infrastructure that caters to the direct supply of drinking water and service water. The requirement of a huge sum is because it requires an integration of technologies that captures the water supply.

A watershed is defined as an area from which rain runoff flows directly into a large stream, river, lake, or pond which has an independent hydrological unit because it provides an optimum use and conservation of soil and water resources. A development of an integrated watershed refers to the development and management of the water resources that achieve higher sustainable production without ecological imbalances because the proper management of watershed restores the ecosystem. One activity that achieves the reduction of surface runoff is by constructing a suitable structure or by changes in land management. Further, the reduction of surface runoff will increase infiltration and help in water conservation.

4. Design of rainwater harvesting using axiomatic design

Rainwater harvesting sustainability requires engineering the rainwater harvesting process and designing it to support demand of increasing population and the financing to enable the development of the infrastructure according to its demand. The design parameters of rainwater harvesting systems includes rain, catchment area (roof, pavement area, storm drains, etc.), conveyance system (gutters, downpipes), storage units or tanks (overground/underground), and distribution system (pipelines, pumps)with the addition of disinfection method such as chlorination and UV (**Table 2**).

The equation used to design based on the rational method is

$$\text{Rainwater Harvested} = \text{Rainfall (mm/year)} \times \text{Catchment area (m)} \times \text{Runoff Coefficient} \tag{1}$$

A water conservation approach can increase the period of water availability and overcome water scarcity through agronomic and engineering procedures. Agronomics or the science that deals with field crop production and soil management has measures that include contour farming, off-season tillage, deep tillage, mulching, and providing vegetative barriers on the contour, which mainly prevent soil erosion and also help in improving soil moisture availability in the watershed.

Type of catchments	Coefficients
Ground surface coverings	0.6–0.8*
• Concrete	0.6–0.9
• The acrylic glass (PMMA)	0.7–0.8*
• Plastic sheeting	0.8–0.9*

**Adapted from Roger S.*

Table 2.
Runoff coefficients.

4.1 What is axiomatic design (AD)?

Suh defines axiomatic design as a design that provides a clear basis to improve the technical design process based on logical and rational thought processes and tools [20]. The AD simplifies the complexity of the modeling and simulation as designers identify what they want to achieve. In the case of rainwater harvesting infrastructure, building a model is identified achievable than creating infrastructure as funding is a challenge with a difficult economy not only in PNG but to many developing countries. With the building of a model, it achieves how accurately it will simulate the design of the rainwater harvesting. The process Axiomatic Design (AD) on infrastructure development of rainwater harvesting is illustrated by Betasolo and Smith [15] in **Figures 5** and **6**.

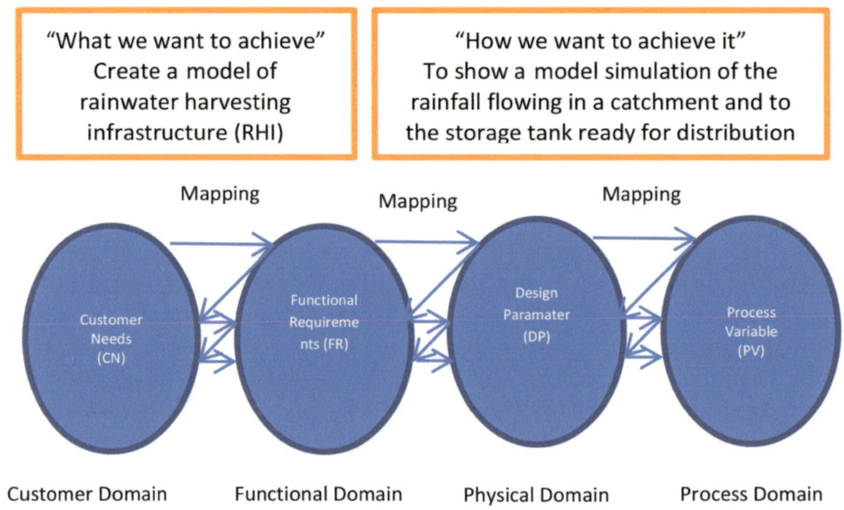

Figure 5.
AD mapping from CN to FR to PD and PV. (Adapted from Betasolo and Smith).

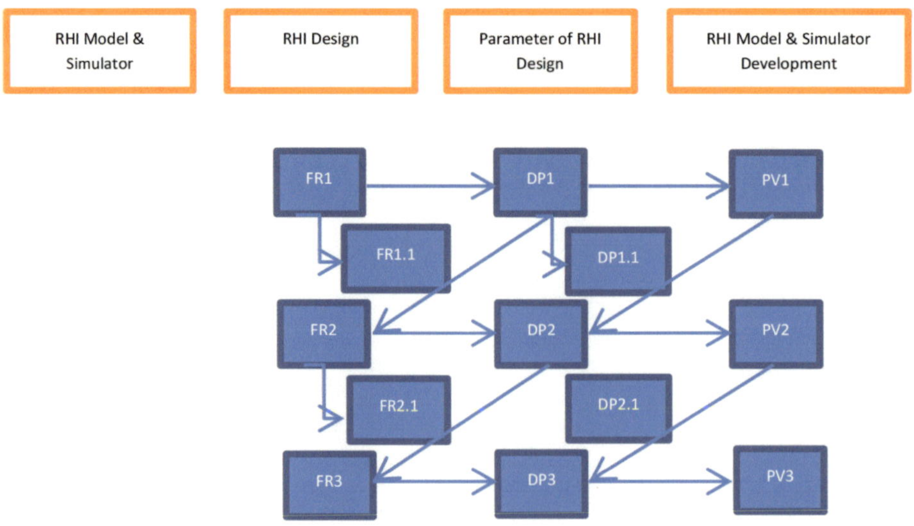

Figure 6.
AD decomposition of FR, PD, and PV. (Adapted from Betasolo and Smith.)

DOI: http://dx.doi.org/10.5772/intechopen.90342

DPs		RHI system	Lightweight and transparent	Coefficient of runoff	Dimension of catchment	Shower or rain	Filter membrane	Tank	Clorination	Outlet
FRs		**DP0**	**DP1**	**DP1.1**	**DP2**	**DP2.1**	**DP3**	**DP4**	**DP5**	**DP6**
FR0	Fabricate an RHI model prototype	x	0	0	0	0	0	0	0	0
FR1	Determine the material to be used	0	x	0	0	0	0	0	0	0
FR1.1	Determine reliability of collecting surface	0	0	x	0	0	0	0	0	0
FR2	Estimate the water to be harvested	0	0	0	x	0	0	0	0	0
FR2.1	Simulate rain (dry and wet)	0	0	0	0	x	0	0	0	0
FR3	Remove dirt and other contamination	0	0	0	0	0	x	0	0	0
FR4	Contain water	0	0	0	0	0	0	x	0	0
FR5	Protect water quality	0	0	0	0	0	0	0	x	0
FR6	Provide point for distribution	0	0	0	0	0	0	0	0	x

Table 3.
Rainwater harvesting infrastructure model prototype design matrix. (Adapted from Betasolo and Smith.)

4.1.1 FR and DP analysis

Table 3 shows the rainwater harvesting infrastructure model prototype design matrix. The design matrix shows a simplified decision where many alternatives and varying criteria are of importance for consideration.

The development of an RHI a requirements for its functionality such as the FR0: Fabricate a model prototype to showcase the RHI system (DP0) which is the design parameter because of the financial constraint to construct the infrastructure. The model prototype will show how the RHI system works and can be used to persuade investor to make the investment to the development of the infrastructure. The functional requirement FR1: Determine the material to be used. The material is affected by the collecting surface reliability (FR1.1). The quality of the surface affects the flow of the rainwater and the amount of rainwater collected. The process of functional requirement and design parameter continues (FR2–FR6 to DP2–DP6) until the requirements are satisfied.

4.2 RHI designing the model prototype

4.2.1 Factors affecting the model prototype

In the creation of a model, there are factors that a designer of RHI should consider. In modeling a rainwater harvesting system, first calculate the amount of rainwater to be collected by the catchment area affected by the nature surface as discussed in Section 3.2 as it relates to the material used in the catchment model prototype or even in actual site in which its slope, dimensions, the storage tank, and the water tightness of the reservoir are set up.

A rainfall catchment system design is composed of five (5) primary parameters such as rainfall pattern, water demand pattern, collection area, storage capacity, and system reliability. The rainfall amount is influenced by the rainfall amount that the area of the catchment is designed. For storage of water collected from the catchment, the size of the tank is based. Therefore, in creating a model prototype, the rainfall simulator included the catchment surface, an inlet canal, a filter compartment, circulation ports, storage tank, and a cleanout outlet as shown in **Figure 7**. To support the movement of the model prototype, an aluminum frame support is used.

A demonstration to final year students was carried out to test the water tightness of the unit and the simulation of rainfall pattern, as shown in **Figure 8**.

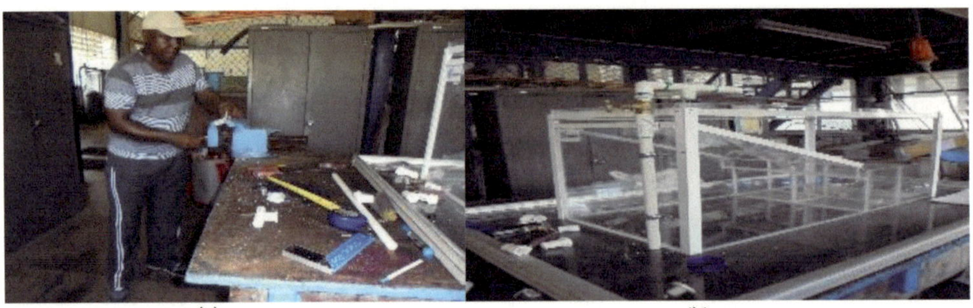

(a) (b)

Figure 7.
(a) RHI model piping system on the making by Carl Smith; (b) the rainwater simulator represented by showerhead system placed at a distance from a rain tray, surface runoff, and the storage tank of RHI model.

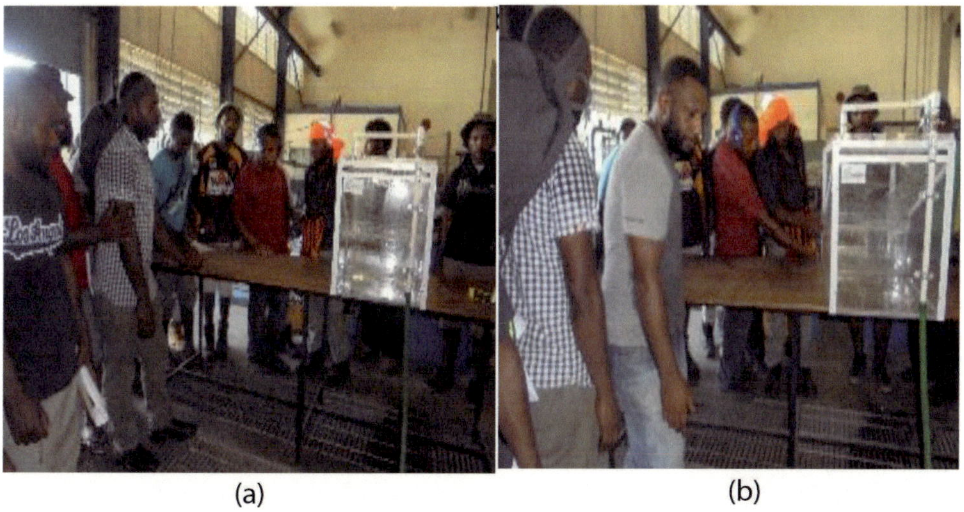

Figure 8.
(a) Test on water tightness of tanks; (b) demonstration of rainwater simulating falling to the catchment area of RHI model.

5. Financing the rainwater harvesting infrastructure

In determining whether RWH is a viable water supply system, the rainfall pattern over the year plays a key role since economy and cost play important criteria in the infrastructure development. Tropical climate with short (1–4 months) dry seasons and high-intensity rainstorms provides the most suitable conditions for water harvesting in Lae City of Papua New Guinea. In addition, rainwater harvesting may also be valuable in wet tropical climates, where the water quantity varies greatly throughout the year. As a general rule, rainfall should be over 50 mm/month for at least half a year or 300 mm/year (unless other sources are extremely scarce) to make RWH environmentally feasible.

An example of an RHI with a catchment area of 3997.1 m^2 from Betasolo and Smith is estimated to cost for one (1) unit of \$220,000.00 (0.6 M in Kina, Papua New Guinea's currency, \$1 = K3) or about \$50/m^2 (K150/m^2). The estimated household population to be served by the prototype is 5415 (the details of the calculation can be found in item 3.0 RHI designing the model of this paper). The infrastructure storage tank can hold about 11,320,500 liters (11.3 M m^3) annually or about 943,375 liters/day (943.4 m^3/day). It provides an approximate annual investment of K0.05/liter (K0.15/m^3). The current price for 1-liter bottled water is K3.5; if this amount is used to calculate for such investment, it will cost a total of \$425,600 (K 1,276,800.00), a savings of about 47%. One of the authors pays \$2/gal (K6/gal) or K1.5/liter for purified drinking water from a vendor.

Household infrastructure is not an ideal infrastructure system in rainwater harvesting due to the high-cost investment that only few can afford. However, for the majority of people, support from the government and private investment is necessary to make the infrastructure possible. Infrastructure finance from private investors and government or a public and private partnership (PPP) model creates opportunity for a design pitch of economically rational financing structures that has a better diversification of risks. The World Bank, ADB, and other similar institutions are some of the few institutions that support financing on such infrastructure.

6. Managing the rainwater harvesting infrastructure for sustainability

Because of the large sum of funds involved in the development of rainwater harvesting infrastructure, a management system should be in place for sustainability. A prototype or a model can be a method to assess performance and lessons learned. For example, rainwater harvesting infrastructure that supports farmers should involve farmers in planning and executing field programs. Ownership of the infrastructure should be channeled to the people who are the beneficiaries. As owners-beneficiaries, responsibility is also shared with the technical advice provider in the management as capabilities to run the rainwater harvesting infrastructure require an expert in handling issues associated to it.

7. Conclusion

The rainwater harvesting infrastructure management is essential especially when dealing with a facility that involves great cost. Understanding of the rainwater harvesting pros and cons is important in the selection of right infrastructure. The design of the infrastructure using an axiomatic design process saves the trial and error, but directly attending to the customer needs and designing it according to the functional requirement coupled with a model prototype show the possibility of the infrastructure to be implemented and investment to flow. Management should start at the beginning of the conceptualization of any infrastructure, to design and financing.

Author details

Mirzi Betasolo* and Carl Smith
Papua New Guinea University of Technology, Lae, Morobe Province, Papua New Guinea

*Address all correspondence to: mirzi.betasolo@pnguot.ac.pg

References

[1] NASA. Hydrologic Cycle [Internet]. 2019. Available from: https://www.nasa.gov/audience/forstudents/5 8/features/Observatorium_Feat_5-8.html [Accessed: May 17, 2019]

[2] ERing, What is rainwater harvesting [Internet]. 2019. Available from: http://www.rainwaterharvesting.org/whatiswh.htm [Accessed: May 17, 2019]

[3] Civil Engineering. Rooftop Rainwater Harvesting [Internet]. Available from: https://www.engineeringcivil.com/roof-top-rain-water-harvesting.html [Accessed: May 17, 2019]

[4] Rainwater Harvesting Systems - Manufacturers, Suppliers ... [Internet]. 2019. Available from: https://www.exportersindia.com/indian-suppliers/rainwater-harvesting-systems.htm[Accessed: May 17, 2019]

[5] Civil Engineering. Research Papers - Page 2 – [Internet]. 2019. Available from: https://www.engineeringcivil.com/theory/research-papers/page/2 [Accessed: May 17, 2019]

[6] Ponce V. Groundwater Utilization and Sustainability [Internet]. 2013. Available from: http://groundwater.sdsu.edu/ [Accessed: July 29, 2013]

[7] Muath A. Assessment of Sustainable Yield of Aquifer [Internet]. 2013. Available from: http://www.hwe.org.ps/Projects/Training/Groundwater%20Wells/presentations/Assessment%20of%20Sustainable%20Yields%20aquifers%20%28SESSION%206%29.pdf [Accessed: July 29, 2013]

[8] EMTV. Communities Receive Tuffa Tanks for Water Supply [Internet]. 2019. Available from: https://emtv.com.pg/communities-receive-tuffa-tanks-for-water-supply/ [Accessed: September 29, 2019]

[9] USGS. Water Science School. The Water in You: Water and the Human Body. [Internet] 2019. Available from: https://www.usgs.gov/special-topic/water-science-school/science/water-you-water-and-human-body?qt-science_center_objects=0#qt-science_center_objects [Accessed: 22 November 2019]

[10] Choo R. The Fog Collectors: Harvesting Water From Thin Air [Internet]. 2018. Available from: https://blogs.ei.columbia.edu/2011/03/07/the-fog-collectors-harvesting-water-from-thin-air/ [Accessed: July 20, 2018]

[11] United Nations Department of Economic & Social Affairs (UNDESA). International Decade for Action "Water for Life". 2005-2015. Available from: www.un.org/waterforlifedecade/scarcity.shtml

[12] Peavey HS, Donald RR, George T. Environmental Engineering. Singapore: McGraw-Hill International Editions; 1985. p. 12

[13] Rogers S. Access to clean water: The Guardians. 2016. [Internet]. Available from: http://www.the guardian.com/news/datablog/2009/mar/03/access-water [Accessed: April 01, 2016]

[14] World Bank. The Independent State of Papua New Guinea: Water, Sanitation, and Hygiene Policy Development in Papua New Guinea. Report No: ACS8481. 2016 March 20. Available from: http://documents.worldbank.org/curated/en/849191468285072764/pdf/ACS84810WP0P1448230Box385243B00PUBLIC0.pdf

[15] World Bank. Climate Change Knowledge Portal. Available from: http://sdwebx.worldbank.org/climateportal/index.cfm?page=downscaled_data_

download&menu=historical. [Accessed: July 29, 2013]

[16] Permanent Culture Now. A Gift From Above-Capturing Rainwater for Green Irrigation. Available from: http://www.permanentculturenow.com/a-gift-from-above-capturing-rainwater-for-green-irrigation/ [Accessed: July 29, 2013]

[17] Betasolo M, Samson G, Anthony B. Design of sustainable use and management of groundwater. In: Morobe Province. Proceedings of the 3rd International Workshop on DCEE 2014, DTU Copenhagen; Denmark. pp. 27-36

[18] Betasolo ML, Carl S. Axiomatic Design process in developing a model prototype rainwater harvesting infrastructure. Journal Title: Procedia CIRP.PROCIR4276, PII:S22182711630974. DOI:10.1016/j.procir.2016.09.004

[19] Worldometers. Papua New Guinea Water. 2019. Available from: https://www.worldometers.info/water/papua_new_guinea_water/

[20] Suh NP. The Principles of Design. New York: Oxford University Press; 2001

Chapter 4

Fluoride in Volcanic Areas: A Case Study in Medical Geology

Diana Paula Silva Linhares, Patrícia Ventura Garcia and Armindo dos Santos Rodrigues

Abstract

Volcanic regions have always attracted many people worldwide because of the high fertility of their soils. However, human proximity to volcanoes can lead to several health problems as consequence of the chronic exposure to the materials released from the volcanic activity. An element often found in elevated concentrations in volcanic regions is fluorine. Although fluoride is recognized to have a beneficial effect on the rate of occurrence of dental caries when ingested in small amounts, its excessive intake results in a widespread but preventable pathological disease called fluorosis. While skeletal fluorosis, the most severe form of fluorosis, requires a chronic exposure to high concentrations of fluoride in water (4–8 mg/L), dental fluorosis occurs after shorter periods of exposure to fluoride in lower concentrations (1.5–2.0 mg/L). In some volcanic regions, where exposure to elevated amounts of fluoride is persistent, biomonitoring programs are fundamental to assess the main sources of exposure and to evaluate the effects of the exposure in resident populations. This chapter aims to cover the main effects of fluoride exposure in humans and discuss the use of a multidisciplinary approach that brings together the geoscience, biomedical, and public health communities to address environmental health problems.

Keywords: fluoride, volcanism, geomedicine, geology, geochemistry, health

1. Introduction

1.1 Definition and physical and chemical properties

Fluorine was discovered by Georgius Agricola in 1529. It is a univalent poisonous gaseous halogen with pale yellow-green color and the most chemically reactive and electronegative of all the elements. It is the 13th most abundant element in the earth's crust and is widely dispersed in nature, almost entirely in the form of fluoride.

Fluoride is an inorganic, monoatomic anion being considered the simplest fluorine anion. It is classified as a weak base, since it only partially associates in solution, but concentrated fluoride is corrosive, and it can attack the skin.

1.2 Geochemistry of fluoride

Fluorine is a naturally occurring chemical substance in the earth's crust where it can be found in rocks, coal, and clay; it is also present in minor quantities in air, water, soil, plants, animals, and humans [1].

The distribution of fluorine in the environment is uneven because of geogenic causes. The most common natural sources of fluorine are fluorite, fluorapatite, and cryolite; as for the anthropogenic sources, these include coal burning, oil refining, steel production, brick-making industries, and phosphatic plant fertilizers, among others [2].

Humans can be exposed to fluoride through food and breathing air, but, considering that the most common sources of fluoride in surface and groundwaters are usually natural, such as the leaching of rocks and dissolution of fluorides from volcanic gases [3], the main source of human exposure, especially in volcanic regions, is drinking water.

1.3 Volcanic environments

Volcanoes emit a variety of gases, both between and during eruptions, including H_2O, CO_2, SO_2, HCl, NH_3, H_2S, and HF, and a few other minor constituents [4, 5]. The volcanic activity represents the main natural persistent source of fluorine that is emitted mostly in the form of HF. Its fraction in volcanic gas emissions is less than 1 ppm and presents an annual global emission of 0.06–6 Tg [4]. Although HF is not of importance in general, during specific events the HF emissions may be extreme and lead to severe environmental contamination with hazards to plants and livestock. According to Halmer et al. [6], the annual global HF volcanic gas input into the atmosphere from 1972 to 2000 was of 0.7–8.6 × 1012 g/yr. For volcanic areas, such as Mt. Etna in Italy or Masaya in Nicaragua, it has been estimated that the passive degassing from these volcanoes accounts for 90% of the volcanic fluorine release. The high amounts of fluorine release in volcanic regions and the natural occurrence of excessive amounts of fluoride in drinking water are associated with acute and chronic fluorosis on grazing animals, due either to direct ingestion of F-rich ashes deposited on the grazing grass or drinking water that are F-contaminated [7]. This problem was first recognized in Iceland, a region with F-rich magmas, by Eiriksson in 1693 after the eruption of Mt. Hekla where this farmer observed deformed teeth in sheep, cattle, and horse calling them "ash-teeth"; later on, also in Iceland, half of the livestock population died in 1783 after Laki eruption that released 42 billion tons of basalt lava and clouds of poisonous HF and SO2 compounds that contaminated the soil [8]. Several cases of chronic fluorosis have been associated to passive degassing in the island of Ambrym in Vanuatu, where it is located one of the most vigorous and persistently degassing volcanoes on Earth; throughout this island, the prevalence of dental fluorosis in children aged 6–18 years ranged between 61 and 96% [9]. In Kenya, situated in East Africa, where the Kenyan Rift is formed by numerous volcanoes, the prevalence of dental fluorosis ranges between 44 and 77% [10].

Considering that, in volcanic regions, fluoride is continuously released and that it can pose a health problem for animals and humans, it can be considered a health risk to the populations inhabiting nearby an active volcano, as it happens in the volcanic islands of the Azores archipelago.

The Azores archipelago (Portugal), located in the North Atlantic Ocean, comprises nine volcanic inhabited islands, located between 36°45′–39°45'N and 24°45′–31°17'W, where the Eurasian, African, and American lithospheric plates meet [11]. Due to its specific formation context, seismicity and volcanism are frequent in the archipelago, resulting in the existence of aquifers formed by the volcanic rocks that erupted during the principal building stage of each volcano. In São Miguel island, the largest of archipelago, formed by three major active central volcanoes (Sete Cidades, Fogo and Furnas), high values of fluoride in the groundwaters and endemic fluorosis in some areas of the island have been reported. In

1993, Lobo measured the fluoride concentration in São Miguel Island springs and observed values ranging from 0.1 to 9.9 mg/L [12], evidencing that in some areas fluoride in drinking water exceeded the WHO maximum level (1.5 mg/L) [13]. In some areas, such as the village of Ribeira Quente, located only 5 km from the caldera of Furnas volcano, most of the inhabitants have visible evidence of dental fluorosis in the permanent dentition, due to raised fluoride levels in the drinking water [14]. More recently, in a cross-sectional study conducted among a sample of students from Ponta Delgada, the largest city of the archipelago, and students from Viseu, a non-fluoridated region, results revealed that the prevalence of dental fluorosis in the students of Ponta Delgada was fourfold higher (15.3 vs. 4.1%) [15]. This tendency is observed through the other islands of the archipelago. In Terceira Island, fluoride content in drinking water above the recommended legal values has been recorded, especially in Praia da Vitória municipality area, where the dental fluorosis prevalence in schoolchildren is of 25% [16]. According to Cordeiro et al. [17], about 98% of the Azores water supply originates in groundwater sources, which is a very important feature to consider, since fluoride content in volcanic aquifers may result from rock leaching processes and from the rising volcanic gases that are dissolved in the groundwaters [18–20]. Another feature important to consider when studying the exposure to fluoride in São Miguel Island is that the only tea plantation in Europe occurs in this island and thus the inhabitants have the frequent habit of drinking tea that also contributes to the exacerbation of the effects of fluoride exposure.

2. Human exposure to fluoride

The main sources of human exposure to fluoride are diet, dental hygiene products, dermal absorption from chemicals or pharmaceuticals, and exposure to industrial emissions. Regarding the exposure by diet, it is recognized that of all the common foodstuffs, tea has one of the highest potentials to increase the daily fluoride intake [21, 22], having a fluoride bioavailability close to 100% [23], similar to the drinking water [24]. Most of the fluoride (about 90%) is absorbed in the gastrointestinal tract after its consumption and distributed through the organism via the bloodstream.

Although fluoride has no recognized essential function in human growth and development, it has a fundamental role in the prevention of caries (tooth decay) [25, 26]. As a result, throughout the world many countries started programs of fluoridation of drinking water and the development of fluoride containing oral care products (toothpastes and mouth rinses) and supplements (fluoride tablets), as public health protective measures against tooth decay.

2.1 Human fluorosis

Fluorosis results of a high consumption of F that may cause chronic fluoride toxicity, being harmful and, sometimes, causing severe poisoning that in the absence of medical treatment, can be lethal. One of the main mechanisms involved in the pathogenesis of fluorosis is an increased oxygen radical generation and lipid peroxidation.

Chronic exposure to high levels of fluoride affects specially the skeleton and teeth which are the prime organs of F retention/accumulation in the human body, while relatively small amounts may be deposited in another calcifying organ, as the pineal gland [27, 28]. The most common pathology in fluoride endemic areas is dental fluorosis, which usually occurs in areas where fluoride exposure concentrations are above 1.5–2.0 mg/L. Dental fluorosis has a progressive outcome [29]: in its initial stages, the teeth develop chalky white patches and become rough, and as time goes by, yellow to dark brown lines may also become visible [28–30] in the teeth.

Skeletal fluorosis results from exposure to fluoride in minimum concentrations of 4–8 mg/L [13] and leads to an increase in bone density, calcification of ligaments, and rheumatic or arthritic pain in joints and muscles, along with stiffness and rigidity of the joints. The early symptoms are severe pain in the spine, joints, and hip area; on time, the muscles in the spine will become calcified, and crippling deformities of the spine and the major joints will occur [31].

Since the dental and skeletal fluorosis are irreversible pathologies, the only way to mitigate its effects is through prevention, by keeping fluoride intake within the safety limits defined by the WHO, such as a maximum that is below 1.5 mg/L of fluoride in drinking water [13].

2.2 Human fluorosis due to volcanic activity

Several cases of endemic fluorosis due to high F concentrations in groundwater have been reported in volcanic areas worldwide, particularly in East Africa, India, and China, where millions of people are affected [32]. The association between volcanic activity and human fluorosis was first established in Kyushu Island, Southwest Japan. Due to the activity of the Aso volcano, fluorosis was known as the "Aso volcano disease" and affected all the population living in the hill's foot [33]. After the recognition of this association between the active volcanism and fluorosis, dental fluorosis has been described in many volcanic areas such as Indonesia [34], Kenya [35], Turkey [36], Tenerife Island (Canary, Spain) [37], and São Miguel Island (Azores, Portugal) [14].

The prevalence of skeletal fluorosis is often underestimated due to the similarity of its symptoms with other skeletal diseases; for instance, in 2005 Weinstein [38] showed that Egil Skallagrimsson, an Icelandic poet and warrior, probably suffered from skeletal fluorosis for being chronically exposed to emissions of volcanic eruptions in Iceland, instead of Paget's disease. Weinstein's study highlights the importance of understanding if chronic exposure to fluoride in volcanic environments may lead to the development of fluorosis.

3. Human biomonitoring

In an attempt to prevent excessive exposure to fluoride, the drinking water concentration standards and guidelines are targeted so that total fluoride intake from all sources does not exceed exposure guidance values [39, 40]. Since fluoride occurs naturally in several sources, the exposure to this element is widespread, and therefore programs to quantify the exposure and its effects in human health are often necessary. In human biomonitoring, measurements of the internal dose are assessed in human biological fluids or tissues, thus integrating fluoride absorbed from all exposure routes [41].

3.1 Urine

The concentration of fluoride in urine is used as a biomarker of recent exposure [22, 42, 43], because urine is the main route of elimination of fluoride. In the adult population, about 50% of absorbed fluoride is deposited in calcified tissues, and the remaining is excreted in the urine [44]. Although urinary fluoride concentrations do not provide a direct measure of fluoride due to variations in urine flow and pH, the studies of urinary fluoride levels are ideal for assessing the intake of fluoride in populations [45]. The measurement of urinary fluoride can be performed by several techniques, such as fluoride ion-selective electrode (FISE), based on the methods described by the National Institute for Occupational Safety and Health (NIOSH) [46], high-performance liquid chromatography (HPLC), ion chromatography spectrometry (IC), and colorimetric methods.

3.2 Fingernails

Nails have been used as biomarkers of acute, sub-chronic, and chronic exposure to fluoride [47, 48] in humans, since in this matrix the fluoride concentration reflects the average level of intake and the plasma concentration over a protracted period, usually 1–2 weeks depending on how often the nails are clipped [49].

Fingernails' fluoride is generally measured with a fluoride ion-selective electrode, applying the method developed by Taves [50] and modified by Whitford [51] after overnight HMDS-facilitated diffusion.

Considering that the fluoride measured in nail clippings represents the fluoride obtained from the systemic circulation, either by secondary concentration or by continuous incorporation, this makes nails a useful biomarker for both sub-chronic (exposure to 1–2 mg/L F) and chronic fluoride exposures (exposure to >2 mg/L F).

4. Medical geology

There are several studies about the occurrence of fluoride in the environment and its relationship to human health spanning a wide variety of disciplines that include the fields of medicine, dentistry, environmental and occupational health, toxicology, environmental geology, petrology, geochemistry, economic geology, hydrogeology, and soil science [52].

For more robust evidence of the relationship between fluoride and human health, studies regarding interdisciplinary approaches and combined methods to establish environmental exposures, health outcomes, and the relationships between them [53] are required, instead of the usual unidirectional approaches. Medical geology is defined as "the science dealing with the relationship between geological factors and health problems in humans, animals and plants" [54, 55], and its interdisciplinary approach brings together geosciences, biomedical, and public health communities. This multidisciplinary association allows the identification of natural and anthropogenic sources of harmful materials in the environment, the understanding of how people are exposed to such materials, and what can be done to minimize or prevent such exposure [56].

Medical geology studies allow to establish the background concentrations in the environment of elements, such as fluoride, identifying the areas with high concentrations of this element from those with low and enabling the modeling of the elemental deposition/uptake in the environment.

4.1 Case studies with a medical geology approach

The effects in human health for excessive exposure to fluoride have been studied worldwide, and exposure guidance values have been established. However, nowadays in many regions of the world, fluorosis continues to be endemic. Considering that volcanic aquifers can promote the occurrence of high F contents in groundwater [57, 58], some studies have determined the health impacts of fluoride exposure in drinking water due to volcanic activity. In Vanuatu the constant low-level basaltic volcanic activity results in a continuous release of fluoride gas, which is reflected in cow rib bones and teeth fluoride content in grazing animals. According to Cronin and Sharp (2002), the possible long-term accumulation of F in the grazing animals results from the consumption of plants F-bearing volcanic ash and drinking F-rich waters (in some areas the fluoride concentration in water reached values up to 2.8 mg/L), which represent potential sources of F causing chronic dental and skeletal fluorosis [59]. Also, in New Zealand in the hydrothermal system of Ruapehu volcano, significant concentrations of soluble F in ashes are leached into the soils and water over longer periods, representing a long-term environmental hazard for the inhabitants of this area [19].

Despite the results evidencing the clear association between volcanic activity and fluoride availability, to act in the mitigation and prevention of fluoride exposure, it is necessary to better understand which are the main routes of exposure, since they can differ according to the region in study. In the specific case of São Miguel Island in the Azores archipelago, Portugal, the main routes of human fluoride exposure are the water and some dietary habits, such as the frequent consumption of tea. In this volcanic island, the groundwater geochemistry is influenced by the dissolution of primary minerals of the volcanic rocks [60] that are naturally enriched in fluoride. Also, the habit of tea consumption is well established in the local communities, because this is the only place in Europe where tea is produced, processed, and commercialized [61] since 1883.

Until 2016, there was no information regarding the health effects of chronic fluoride exposure in the inhabitants of this island; although in some studies the authors have identified anomalous values of fluoride in water [12] and clear signals of dental fluorosis in humans [14] and animals [62], none was focused on estimating the effects of the exposure to fluoride in humans. To identify the sources of fluoride in the environment and to assess the effects of the exposure in São Miguel Island inhabitants, studies in medical geology have been developed. In the study by Linhares et al. [63], it was observed that even with modern water treatment systems, there are areas in the island of São Miguel that have fluoride concentrations in water slightly above the recommended legal values. Therefore, these authors developed a study that investigated if urine and nail clippings had sensitivity and/or utility for biomonitoring human population from different age classes that are chronically exposed to fluoride; a positive correlation was found between the fluoride daily intake and fluoride content in children urine, and in adults and children nail clippings, revealing that nail clippings are a more reliable biomarker of chronic exposure to fluoride than urine for populations of different age classes (children vs. adults).

Considering that within the residents of this island, the tea consumption is a well-established habit in adults and children and that tea is a fluoride-bioconcentrating plant, another study was developed in 2017 by Linhares et al. to assess the exposure of humans to fluoride intake through tea infusion consumption [64]. The authors concluded that the Azorean tea brands had higher fluoride content than other international brands. The higher concentration of fluoride in the Azorean tea brands is related to the fact that the soils of the Azores archipelago originate from modern volcanic materials that have evolved under the humid and moderate Atlantic climate, classified as Andosols [65], being naturally enriched in fluoride. With mean results of 3.53 mg/L of fluoride in tea infusions, several concerns regarding the consumption of tea, especially in children, were raised by this study, since by consuming tea the daily intake of fluoride could easily overcome the recommended daily values [64]. This work evidenced that in areas where tea consumption is habitual in all ages and where fluoride content in drinking water exceeds the legislated values, the upper limit threshold for the average fluoride daily intake can be easily exceeded only by tea drinking, contributing to the development of fluorosis in these areas. In this paper, the authors also point out the importance of considering the concentration of fluoride in the water used to make tea.

More recently, Linhares et al. [66] carried a fieldwork using mice (*Mus musculus*) collected in Furnas village (a village located inside the caldera of Furnas volcano, an area where volcanic activity is marked by active fumarolic fields, hot and cold CO2-rich springs, and soil diffuse degassing phenomena [67, 68]) to assess the risk of skeletal fluorosis from the environmental exposure to fluoride in hydrothermal areas. Results showed that mice from Furnas village had higher concentrations of fluoride in bones than mice from an area without volcanic activity [66]. These results reinforce that chronic exposure to fluoride may lead to the development of not only dental fluorosis but also of skeletal fluorosis, which can be misdiagnosed as rheumatism and arthrosis [38], pinpointing the fact that elderly people living chronically exposed to volcanic environments can also suffer from undiagnosed skeletal fluorosis.

5. Risk management

The excessive intake of fluoride and its role on the development of human fluorosis is well known; despite this, fluorosis still occurs in several parts of the world. It continues to show up, not only in the Third World countries, due to the population's lack of choice in their sources of drinking water and food, but also in developed countries, because of fluoridation of the public drinking water, private water supplies, dietary choices, dental products, industrial emissions, and/or occupational exposure. Adding to all these sources of exposure, we must also consider the exposure to fluoride due to natural events, such as volcanic activity, which affects many persons in several regions worldwide.

Since fluorosis, dental and skeletal, can impact upon the biological and psychosocial dimensions of health, it is urgent to work on the prevention and mitigation of human exposure to fluoride. According to the main sources of exposure, the actions that can be taken to address this issue are defluoridation of existing water supplies and/or the establishment of an alternative low-fluoride water source [13]; the modification of rainwater harvesting practices; changes in dietary habits, specifically regarding tea consumption; and an adequate use of dental products.

Nonetheless, multidisciplinary epidemiological studies, gathering areas such geochemistry, epidemiology, and ecotoxicology, are still required since they provide adequate insights regarding dose-response relationship and detailed information about the areas that are naturally fluoride rich. This will assist and guide authorities implementing environmental remediation decisions and developing public health planning and response efforts to reduce fluoride-related health problems.

6. Conclusions

In the Azores, human exposure to fluoride can easily reach values above the recommended guidelines. The most common factors that contribute to an excessive concentration of this element are groundwater naturally enriched in fluoride and consumption of tea. Results from several studies evidence that the chronic exposure to elevated fluoride concentrations contributes not only to the development of dental fluorosis but also, in more severe cases, to the development of skeletal fluorosis.

Considering that water consumption is the most important, but not the only exposure pathway to fluoride, it is fundamental to implement multidisciplinary biomonitoring studies combined with a medical geology approach. This type of strategy identifies harmful geologic agents and determines the conditions of exposure that promote deteriorating health status, providing the necessary knowledge to track a wide range of environmentally and naturally induced health issues such as fluorosis.

Conflict of interest

All the authors state that they have no conflict of interest.

Author details

Diana Paula Silva Linhares[1,2*], Patrícia Ventura Garcia[1,3] and Armindo dos Santos Rodrigues[1,2]

1 Faculty of Sciences and Technology, University of the Azores, Ponta Delgada, Portugal

2 IVAR, Institute of Volcanology and Risks Assessment, University of the Azores, Ponta Delgada, Portugal

3 cE3c, Centre for Ecology, Evolution and Environmental Changes, and Azorean Biodiversity Group, University of the Azores, Ponta Delgada, Portugal

*Address all correspondence to: diana.ps.linhares@uac.pt

References

[1] Agency for Toxic Substances and Disease Registry (ATSDR). Toxicological Profile for Fluorides, Hydrogen Fluoride and Fluorine. Atlanta, GA: U.S. Department of Health and Human Services, Public Health Service; 2003

[2] Dey S, Giri B. Fluoride fact on human health and health problems: A review. Medical & Clinical Reviews. 2015;**2**:2

[3] Garcia MG, Borgnino L. Chapter 1: Fluoride in the context of the environment. In: Preedy VR (ed) Fluorine: Chemistry, Analysis, Function and Effects. London: The Royal Society of Chemistry; 2015. pp. 3-21

[4] Symonds RB, Rose WI, Reed MH. Contribution of Cl- and F-bearing gases to the atmosphere by volcanoes. Nature. 1988;**334**:415-418

[5] Giggenbach WF. Chemical composition of volcanic gases. In: Scarpa RIS, Tilling RI, editors. Monitoring and Mitigation of Volcano Hazards. Heidelberg: Springer; 1996. pp. 221-256

[6] Halmer MM, Schmincke HU, Graf HF. The annual volcanic gas input into the atmosphere, in particular into the stratosphere: A global data set for the past 100 years. Journal of Volcanology and Geothermal Research. 2002;**115**:511-528

[7] D'Alessandro W. Human fluorosis related to volcanic activity: A review. Environmental Toxicology Transaction: Biomedicine and Health. 2006;**10**:21-30

[8] Fridriksson S. Fluoride problems following volcanic eruption. In: Shupe JL, Peterson HB, Leone NC, editors. Fluorides—Effect on Vegetation, Animals and Humans. UT: Pearagon Press; 1983. pp. 339-344

[9] Allibone R, Cronin SJ, Charley DT, et al. Dental fluorosis linked to degassing of Ambrym volcano, Vanuatu: A novel exposure pathway. Environmental Geochemistry and Health. 2012;**34**:155

[10] Kaimenyi TJ. Oral health in Kenya. International Dental Journal. 2004;**54**(6):378

[11] Searle R. Tectonic pattern of the Azores spreading Centre and triple junction. Earth and Planetary Science Letters. 1980;**51**:415-434

[12] Lobo M. Contribuição para o estudo físico-químico e microbiológico da água para consumo humano do arquipélago dos Açores. Universidade dos Açores, Departamento de Ciências Agrárias; 1993

[13] World Health Organization (WHO). Guidelines for Drinking-Water Quality: Recommendations. 3rd ed. Geneva: WHO Press; 2004

[14] Baxter P, Baubron J, Coutinho R. Health hazards and disaster potential of ground gas emissions at Furnas volcano, São Miguel, Azores. Journal of Volcanology and Geothermal Research. 1999;**92**:95-106

[15] Arrimar A. Prevalência de cárie dentária e fluorose dentária numa amostra de crianças e adolescentes de um meio com água fluoretada (Ponta Delgada) e de um meio sem água fluoretada (Viseu)-Estudo piloto. Universidade Católica portuguesa, Centro Regional das beiras—Pólo de Viseu; 2012

[16] Costa S. Avaliação de Fluoretos na Água de Consumo do Concelho da Praia da Vitória (ilha Terceira, Açores) e suas Consequências a Nível da Saúde Pública. Universidade dos Açores, Departamento de Ciências Agrárias—Mestrado de Engenharia e Gestão de Sistemas de Água. 2013

[17] Cordeiro S, Coutinho R, Cruz JV. Fluoride content in drinking water supply in São Miguel volcanic island (Azores, Portugal). Science of the Total Environment. 2012;**432**:23-36

[18] Aiuppa A, Bellomo S, Brusca L, D'Alessandro W, Federico C. Natural and anthropogenic factors affecting groundwater quality of an active volcano (Mt. Etna, Italy). Applied Geochemistry. 2003;**18**:863-882

[19] Cronin SJ, Neall VE, Lecointre JA, Hedley MJ, Loganathan P. Environmental hazards of fluoride in volcanic ash: A case study from Ruapehu volcano, New Zealand. Journal of Volcanology and Geothermal Research. 2003;**121**:271-291

[20] Flaathen T, Gislason S. The effect of volcanic eruptions on the chemistry of surface waters: The 1991 and 2000 eruptions of Mt. Hekla, Iceland. Journal of Volcanology and Geothermal Research. 2007;**164**:293-316

[21] National Research Council. Review of Fluoride in Drinking Water, U.S. Washington, DC, USA: The National Academic Press; 2006

[22] World Health Organization. Fluorine and Fluoride, Environmental Health Criteria 36. Geneva, Switzerland: World Health Organization; 1984

[23] Tokalıoğlu S, Kartal S, Sahin U. Determination of fluoride in various samples and some infusions using a fluoride selective electrode. Turkish Journal of Chemistry. 2004;**28**:203-211

[24] Rao GS. Dietary intake and bioavailability of fluoride. Annual Review of Nutrition. 1984;**4**:115-136

[25] Petersen PE, Lennon MA. Effective use of fluorides for the prevention of dental caries in the 21st century: The WHO approach. Community Dentistry and Oral Epidemiology. 2004;**32**:319-321

[26] Buzalaf MA, Pessan JP, Honorio HM, Cate JM. Mechanisms of action of fluoride for caries control. Monographs in Oral Science. 2011;**22**:97-114

[27] Doull J, Boekelheide K, Farishian BG, Isaacson RL, Klotz JB, Kumar JV, et al. Committee on Fluoride in Drinking Water, Board on Environmental Studies and Toxicology, Division on Earth and Life Studies, National Research Council of the National Academies. Fluoride in Drinking Water: A Scientific Review of EPA's Standards. Washington, DC: The National Academies Press; 2006. pp. 181-204

[28] Kumar N, Bansal N, Sharma SK. Determination of fluoride status in ground water of Rajasthan. International Journal of Pharmaceutical, Chemical and Biological Sciences. 2014;**4**:576-592

[29] Cao SR, Li YF. The evaluation of indoor air quality in areas of endemic fluorosis caused by coal combustion. In: Proceedings of the XIX Conference of the International Society for Fluoride Research, Kyoto, Japan. Kyoto: Department of Hygiene and Public Health, Osaka Medical College; 1992. p. 38

[30] World Health Organization (WHO). Guideline for Drinking Water Quality. 2rd ed. Geneva: WHO Press; 1997

[31] Annaduraia TS, Rengasamya KJ, Sundaramb R, Munusamy PA. Incidence and effects of fluoride in Indian natural ecosystem: A review. Advances in Applied Science Research. 2014;**5**:173-185

[32] Brindha K, Elango L. Fluoride in groundwater: Causes, implications and mitigation measures. In: Monroy SD,

editor. Fluoride Properties, Applications and Environmental Management. Hauppauge, Nova: Nova Science Publishers; 2011. p. 111-136

[33] Kawahara S. Odontological observations of Mt. Aso-volcano disease. Fluoride. 1971;**4**:172-175

[34] Heikens A, Sumatri S, Bergen M, Widianarko B, Fokkert L, Leeuwen K, et al. The impact of the hyperacid Ijen crater Lake: Risks of excess fluoride to human health. Science of the Total Environment. 2005;**36**(1-3):56-59

[35] Wambu EW, Muthakia GK. High fluoride water in the Gilgil area of Nakuru County, Kenya. Fluoride. 2011;**44**(1):37-41

[36] Oruc N. Occurrence and problems of high fluoride waters in Turkey: An overview. Environmental Geochemistry and Health. 2008;**30**(4):315-323

[37] Hardisson A, Rodriguez MI, Burgos A, Flores LD, Gutierrez R, Varela H. Fluoride levels in publicly supplied and bottled drinking water in the island of Tenerife, Spain. The Bulletin of Environmental Contamination and Toxicology. 2001;**67**(2):163-170

[38] Weinstein P. Palaeopathology by proxy: The case of Egil's bones. Journal of Archaeological Science. 2005;**32**:1077-1082

[39] Health Canada. Guidelines for Canadian Drinking Water Quality: Guideline Technical Document—Fluoride. Water, Air and Climate Change Bureau, Healthy Environments and Consumer Safety Branch, Health Canada, Ottawa, Ontario. (Catalogue No. H128-1/11-647E-PDF). 2010

[40] United States Environmental Protection Agency (USEPA). Fluoride: Dose-Response Analysis for Non-cancer Effects. 820-R-10-019. Health and Ecological Criteria Division, Office of Water, Washington, D.C. 2010

[41] Saravanabhavan G, Werry K, Walker M, Haines D, Malowany M, Khoury C. Human biomonitoring reference values for metals and trace elements in blood and urine derived from the Canadian health measures survey 2007-2013. International Journal of Hygiene and Environmental Health. 2017;**220**:189-200

[42] Villa A, Anabalon M, Zohouri V, Maguire A, Franco AM, Rugg-Gunn A. Relationships between fluoride intake, urinary fluoride excretion and fluoride retention in children and adults: An analysis of available data. Caries Research. 2010;**44**:60-68

[43] Rugg-Gunn AJ, Villa AE, Buzalaf MR. Contemporary biological markers of exposure to fluoride. Monographs in Oral Science. 2011;**22**:37-51

[44] Hodge HC, Smith FA, Gedalia I. Excretion of fluorides. In: Fluorides and Human Health, World Health Organization Monograph Series No. 59. Geneva: WHO; 1970. pp. 141-161

[45] Aylward LL, Hays SM, Vezina A, Deveau M, St-Amand A, Nong A. Biomonitoring equivalents for interpretation of urinary fluoride. Regulatory Toxicology and Pharmacology. 2015;**72**:158-167

[46] NIOSH (National Institute for Occupational Safety and Health). Fluoride in urine. In: Manual of Analytical Methods. 3rd ed. Vol. II. Washington DC: U.S. Department of Health and Human Services; 1984

[47] Czarnowski W, Krechniak J. Fluoride in urine, hair and nails of phosphate fertilizer workers. British Journal of Industrial Medicine. 1990;**47**:349-351

[48] Feskanich D, Owusu W, Hunter DJ, Willett WC, Ascherio A, Spiegelman D, et al. Use of toenail fluoride levels as an indicator for the risk of hip and forearm

fractures in women. Epidemiology. 1998;**9**:412-416

[49] Whitford GM. Monitoring fluoride exposure with fingernail clippings. Schweizer Monatsschrift für Zahnmedizin. 2005;**115**:685-689

[50] Taves DR. Determination of submicromolar concentrations of fluoride in biological samples. Talanta. 1968;**15**:1015-1023

[51] Whitford GM. In: Myers HM, editor. The Metabolism and Toxicity of Fluoride. Basel: S Karger; 1996. pp. 25-29 and 86-90

[52] Ozsvath DL. Fluoride and environmental health: A review. Reviews in Environmental Science and Bio/Technology. 2009;**8**(1):59-79

[53] Wardrop NA, Le Blonde JS. Assessing correlations between geological hazards and health outcomes: Addressing complexity in medical geology. Environment International. 2015;**84**:90-93

[54] Selinus O. Medical geology: Method, theory and practice. In: Bobrowsky PT, editor. Geoenvironmental Mapping: Methods, Theory and Practice. New York: A.A. Balkema; 2002. pp. 473-496

[55] Finkelman RB, Skinner HCW, Plumlee GS, Bunnell JE. Medical geology. Geotimes. 2001;**46**(11):20-23

[56] Sunitha V, Reddy MR. Medical geology: A globally emerging discipline. Advances in Bioresearch. 2012;**3**(2):12-20

[57] Rango T, Bianchini G, Beccaluva L, Ayenew T, Colombani N. Hydrogeochemical study in the main Ethiopian rift: New insights to the source and enrichment mechanism of fluoride. Environmental Geology. 2009;**58**:109-118

[58] Vivona R, Preziosi E, Madé B, Giuliano G. Occurrence of minor toxic elements in volcanic-sedimentary aquifers: A case study in Central Italy. Hydrogeology Journal. 2007;**15**:1183-1196

[59] Cronin SJ, Sharp DS. Environmental impacts on health from continuous volcanic activity at Yasur (Tanna) and Ambrym, Vanuatu. International Journal of Environmental Health Research. 2002;**12**:109-123

[60] Cruz JV. Groundwater and volcanoes: Examples from the Azores archipelago. Environmental Geology. 2003;**44**:343-355

[61] Baptista J, Lima E, Paiva L, Andrade AL, Alves MG. Comparison of Azorean tea Theanine to teas from other origins by HPLC/DAD/FD. Effect of fermentation, drying temperature, drying time and shoot maturity. Food Chemistry. 2012;**132**:2181-2187

[62] Cunha L, Zanon V, Amaral A, Ferreira J, Rodrigues A. Altered inorganic composition of enamel and dentin in mice teeth chronically exposed to an enriched mineral environment at Furnas, São Miguel (Azores). Arquipelago: Life and Marine Sciences. 2011;**28**:33-37

[63] Linhares D, Garcia P, Amaral L, Ferreira T, Cury J, Vieira W, et al. Sensitivity of two biomarkers for biomonitoring exposure to fluoride in children and women: A study in a volcanic area. Chemosphere. 2016;**155**:614-620

[64] Linhares D, Garcia P, Ferreira T, Rodrigues A. Safety evaluation of fluoride content in tea infusions consumed in the Azores - a volcanic region with water springs naturally enriched in fluoride. Biological Trace Element Research. 2017;**179**: 158-164

[65] Soil Survey Staff. Keys to Soil Taxonomy. 12th ed. Washington, DC: USDA Natural Resources Conservation Service; 2014

[66] Linhares D, Camarinho R, Garcia PV, Rodrigues AR. Mus musculus bone fluoride concentration as a useful biomarker for risk assessment of skeletal fluorosis in volcanic areas. Chemosphere. 2018;**205**:540-544

[67] Cruz J, Coutinho RM, Carvalho MR, Oskarsson N, Sigurdur RG. Chemistry of waters from Furnas volcano, Sao Miguel, Azores: Fluxes of volcanic carbon dioxide and leached material. Journal of Volcanology and Geothermal Research. 1999;**92**:151-167

[68] Ferreira T, Gaspar JL, Viveiros F, Marcos M, Faria C, Sousa F. Monitoring of fumarole discharge and CO_2 soil degassing in the Azores: Contribution to volcanic surveillance and public health risk assessment. Annals of Geophysics. 2005;**48**:4-5

Chapter 5

Biophysical and Economic Factors of Climate Change Impact Chain in the Agriculture Sector of ECOWAS

Calvin Atewamba and Edward R. Rhodes

Abstract

The chapter assesses key biophysical and economic factors of climate change impact chain in the agriculture sector of the Economic Community of West African States (ECOWAS), mainly within the decade following the launching of the Comprehensive Africa Agricultural Development Programme (CAADP) and Maputo Accord. This is done through a review of literature and analysis of data mainly from international databases. We find that land resources for agricultural production are substantial, but land degradation and land productivity are serious problems, particularly in the context of climate change. Although the region has experienced unprecedented growth, financing agricultural development is still an issue. Developing quality infrastructure and stimulating agricultural trade may provide a win-win strategy to build resilience to climate change and strengthen economic development. The economics of adaptation to climate change in the agricultural sector of ECOWAS has mainly focused on the magnitude of costs and returns on country-wide and technology-specific measures. There is a need, however, to integrate biophysical and economic factors of climate change impact chain in sound analytical frameworks to provide "multi-metric" considerations of non-monetary and nonmarket measures, risks, inequities, and behavioral biases in addressing climate change.

Keywords: agriculture, climate adaptation, CAADP, ECOWAS, land degradation, Maputo accord, climate change, infrastructure, trade, climate finance

1. Introduction

Four major agroecological zones span the Economic Community of West African States (ECOWAS) region: these are the Sahelian, Sudan Savannah, Guinea Savannah, and Forest zone. At a broader level, ECOWAS has been grouped into a Gulf of Guinea zone and a Sudano-Sahelian zone based on geographical and climatic homogeneity [1]. All the Gulf of Guinea countries have shorelines with the Atlantic Ocean. The Sudano-Sahelian zone as a whole experiences a hotter and drier climate than the Gulf of Guinea zone. The countries in the former zone are Benin, Cote d'Ivoire, Ghana, Guinea, Guinea-Bissau, Liberia, Nigeria, Sierra Leone, and Togo. Burkina Faso, Cape Verde, the Gambia, Mali, Niger, and Senegal are in the latter zone. While the savannah spreads through both zones, the humid forest agro-ecology is mainly restricted to the Gulf of Guinea (**Figure 1**). The United Nations classified 11 of the 15 countries as least developed based on human resources, poverty level, and economic vulnerability. The exceptions were Ghana, Nigeria, Cote d'Ivoire, and Cape Verde [2]. However, because of its size, natural resources, and importance of agriculture in the economies, ECOWAS has a potential of contributing significantly to world trade, food security, and carbon storage.

Agriculture is the key sector of ECOWAS economies and the one that supports nearly 60% of the region population. The Comprehensive Africa Agriculture Development Programme (CAADP) and the declaration on agriculture and food security by the African Union commonly known as the "Maputo Accord" of 2003 promoted investment for the expansion of the area under sustainable land and water management, increased food supply and agricultural research, and technology dissemination in sub-Saharan Africa and the adoption of a policy of allocating at least 10% of annual national budgets to agriculture and attainment of 6% annual growth in the agriculture sector. The achievement of these goals is under threat from climate change, bearing in mind that the vulnerability of countries in ECOWAS to climate change is among the highest in the world [4]. Therefore, a critical challenge facing the region is how to feed an expected population of around 600 million by 2050 while simultaneously reducing and responding to climate change. There is a growing number of studies analyzing how agricultural production and commodity markets need to be adjusted to promote interregional balance in agricultural production and food security in response to climate change [5–9]. However, the uncertainties with regard to climate change impacts on agriculture remain considerable, and climate change impacts on food security are even less clear. The development of appropriate adaptation and mitigation measures to respond to or combat climate change is dependent on the knowledge of the climate change impacts as well as the nature and trends of the climate change impact chain factors.

The objective of this chapter is to broadly assess at the regional and zonal levels key biophysical and economic factors of the climate change impact chain in

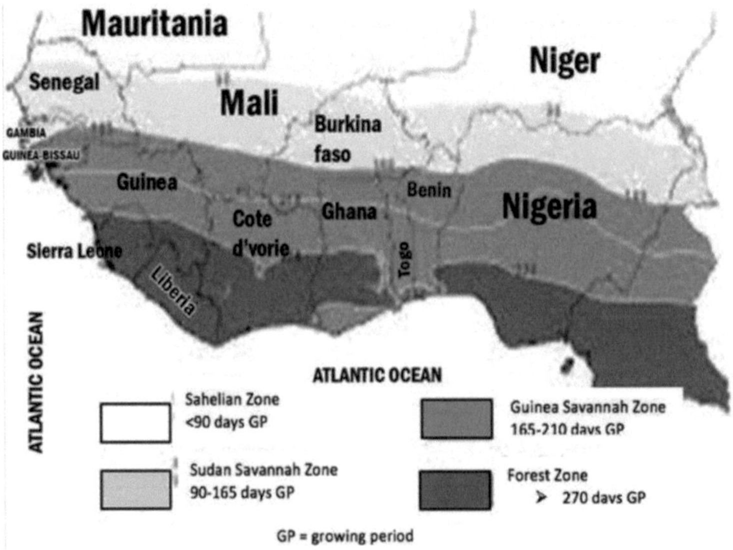

Figure 1.
Location of ECOWAS member states. Source: Adapted from [3].

ECOWAS, especially within a decade after the CAADP and the Maputo Accord, and the economics of adaptation in the crop's subsector. The assessment consists of an analysis of data from international databases and sources and information from other studies. Country national level data on land use, crop production, and yield for 2003 and 2013 are taken mainly from FAO and the World Bank databases and sources. Sums, means, ranges, and percentages are computed.

The remainder of the chapter is organized as follows. In Section 2, we underline the conceptual framework of climate change impact chain in the agriculture sector. Section 3 presents the biophysical factors, mainly land resources, land use, land degradation, and crop production. The economic factors are analyzed in Section 4, where we discussed how growth, inflation, infrastructure, and trade may shape the impacts of climate change on the agricultural sector of ECOWAS. In Section 5, we investigate the current knowledge on the economics of adaptation to climate change and raise the concern of integrating biophysical and economic factors to inform decision-making. Section 6 concludes and makes some remarks for further research.

2. Conceptual framework of climate change impact chain in the agriculture sector

The extent to which climate change affects the agriculture sector and food security depends on the flow of impacts from the environmental system to the economic system through biophysical and social systems that define the agriculture sector. The chain of climate change impacts can be conceptualized as follows (**Figure 2**).

Global warming manifests itself as increasing global mean air and ocean surface temperatures, which directly affect the local environmental system of agriculture, including climate, hydrology, and soil. Changes in the environmental system affect land use, crop yield, and production, which define the biophysical system of

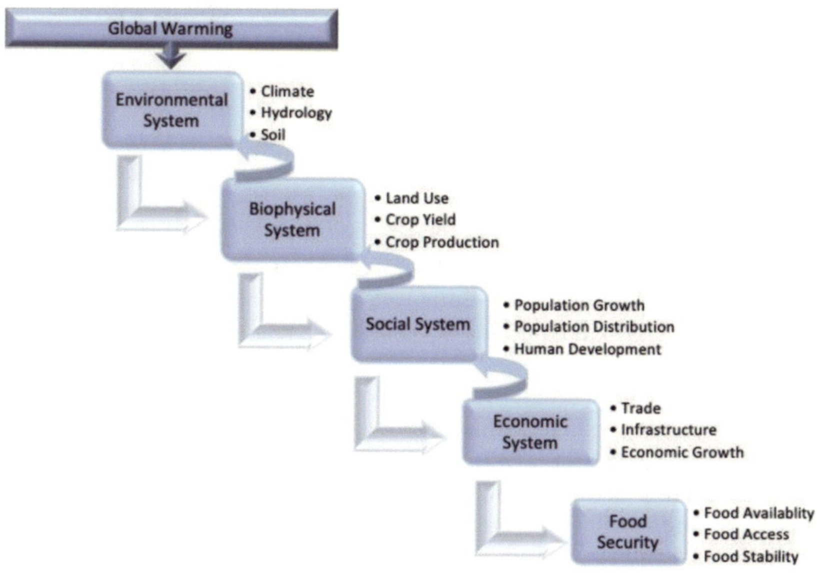

Figure 2.
Climate change impact chain in the agriculture sector.

agriculture. The social system (population growth and distribution, human development) and the economic system (economic growth, trade, infrastructure) define the adaptive capacity of the agriculture sector to manage the changes in the biophysical system in order to guarantee food availability, access, and stability for the population. The resilience of these systems to the wave of climate-induced shocks defines the extent and the magnitude of climate change impact on the agriculture and food security. Indeed, these systems can either moderate or exacerbate the wave of climate-induced chocks on agriculture and food security. For example, if the biophysical system is vulnerable to climate-induced chocks, while the economic system is resilient, then the impact of climate change on agriculture and food security will be reduced.

Mapping the climate change impact chain in the agriculture sector may allow researchers and policy makers to understand the impacts of climate change and identify opportunities and challenges to reduce these impacts on agriculture and food security. In the following sections, we will investigate the biophysical and economic systems of the climate change impact chain in the agriculture sector of ECOWAS.

3. Biophysical factors: land resources, land use, land degradation, and crop production

3.1 Land resources, land use, and land degradation

The total surface area of ECOWAS is 504 million hectares made up of 207 million hectares in the Gulf of Guinea and 297 million hectares in the Sudano-Sahelian [10]. Total cultivable land area for the 15 ECOWAS countries is 196 million hectares out of which 130 million hectares were in the Gulf of Guinea and 66 million hectares in the Sudano-Sahelian zone [1]. Information on land use in 2003 and 2013 are shown in **Table 1**; some aspects were discussed by [11] who concluded that the situation is, in general, deteriorating.

The proportion of protected lands increased in both the Gulf of Guinea and Sudano-Sahelian zones probably indicating responsiveness by governments to global concerns for the preservation of natural resources. This contrasts with a decrease from 19.5 to 13.8% over the same period in protected lands in high-income countries [9, 13]. Lands under arable plus permanent crops were 31.8 and 9.7% in the Gulf of Guinea and Sudano-Sahelian zones, respectively, in 2003 and 33–11% in 2013. Land under arable crops increased to a much greater extent in the Sudano-Sahelian than the Gulf of Guinea. Overall, land under arable crops in ECOWAS increased by 7.3%. Area under permanent crops increased more in the Sudano-Sahelian than in the Gulf of Guinea, with an average increase of 10.5% for ECOWAS. Arable land plus permanent crop lands as a proportion of total land was almost the same in 2003 and in 2013 in the Gulf of Guinea. In the Sudano-Sahelian, there was a small increase from 9.7 in 2003 to 11.3% in 2013. For ECOWAS as a whole, it was 18.7% in 2003 and 20.2% in 2013.

These findings suggest a high proportion of land reserves for agricultural production and variability between zones. However, it would have been more meaningful to express arable plus permanent croplands as a percentage of cultivable land, but the definition of cultivable land lacks clarity. According to [1] "cultivable area is an area of land potentially fit for cultivation. This term may or may not include part or all of the forests and rangeland. Assumptions made in assessing cultivable land vary from country to country. In this (FAO) survey, national figures have been used whenever available, despite possible large discrepancies in computation methods."

Land use	Gulf of Guinea	Sudano-Sahelian	ECOWAS	Gulf of Guinea	Sudano-Sahelian	ECOWAS
	2003	2003	2003	2013	2013	2013
Protected land (percentage of total land)						
Mean	4.8	7.4	5.7	18.5	13.3	16.8
Range	0.7–11.4	2.3–11.6	0.7–11.6	2.4–27.1	4.4–24.2	2.4–27.1
Arable crop land (ha × 1000)						
Total	51,367	28,371	79,738	52,434	33,106	85,540
Range	270–35,000	47–14,050	47–35,000	300–34,000	55–16,800	55–34,000
Permanent crop land (ha × 1000)						
Total	14,257	322	14,579	15,685	427	16,112
Range	130–6450	2–145	2–6450	165–6500	4–150	4–6500
Arable + permanent crop land (percentage of total land)						
Total	31.8	9.7	18.74	33.0	11.3	20.2
Range	6.4–45.9	5.0–30.5	5.0–45.9	7.3–52.2	5.4–44.5	5.4–52.2
Forests (ha × 1000)						
Total	52,903	22,336	75,239	47,717	20,436	68,153
Range						
Forests (percentage of total land)						
Total	25.6	7.5	15.0	23.1	6.9	13.5
Range	7.9–74.7	1.0–45.4	1.0–74.7	4.2–71.1	0.9–43.3	0.9–71.1
Carbon stocks in forests (million t)						
Total	5874	834	6708	5264	770	6034
Range	38–1841	3.7–352	3.7–1841	20–1839	3.9–336	3.9–1839

Source: Author's calculations from [10–12].

Table 1.
Land use: areas under arable and permanent crops and carbon storage in forests in ECOWAS.

Research is therefore needed on reliably estimating cultivable land to facilitate the assessment of key factors controlling climate change impacts.

Area under forests declined at the rate of 9.8 and 8.5% in the Gulf of Guinea and Sudano-Sahelian, respectively. Overall, there was a 9.4% decline in area under forests in ECOWAS over 10 years (**Table 1**). The decline in the Sudano-Sahelian zone may, however, not be uniform because the conversion of biomass into forest has taken place in the Sudano-Sahelian zone [15]. The increase in arable area and decrease in area under forests in ECOWAS associated with the release of carbon to the atmosphere would contribute to land degradation.

The estimated carbon stocks in forests of ECOWAS (**Table 1**) were substantial (6708 million t in 2003 and 6034 million t in 2013) but significantly greater in the Gulf of Guinea, where forests predominate, than the Sudano-Sahelian. The variation of carbon stocks with agroecosystems as measured in the field and laboratory [16] showed that for mangrove ecosystems, roots and soil together accounted for about 86% of the total ecosystem carbon stocks (463 and 1382 Mg C ha^{-1} in the low mangroves of semiarid Senegal and in the tall mangroves of humid Liberia, respectively).

ECOWAS countries have experienced significant land degradation [15, 17]. Based on land area data of the World Bank [10, 14] and areas of degraded land [17], it is estimated that up to 644,000 km^2 (31%) of lands in the Gulf of Guinea and 1,124,000 km^2 (38%) of lands in the Sudano-Sahelian zone and 1,768,000 km^2 (35%) of lands in ECOWAS were severely to very severely degraded by 2000. Nkonya et al. [18], however, reported a lower but still important rate of 19% of lands excluding deserts for Niger. The primary causes of land degradation in ECOWAS are deforestation, agriculture, conversion of grasslands to croplands, and overgrazing [18, 19]. Deforestation in ECOWAS is associated with slash and burn agriculture as well as with fuelwood, charcoal, and timber production to meet basic livelihood needs of small-holder farmers and boost incomes of commercial enterprises. Moussa et al. [19] estimate that more than 60% of carbon dioxide emission in Africa is due to deforestation and land degradation. Land reclamation to combat degradation is therefore a climate change adaptation option requiring financing by governments and their international development partners.

3.2 Crop production

The FAO database on crop production is available on the basis of country and not on farming systems or agroecological zones (AEZ). Nevertheless, it is well known that millet and sorghum are the traditional cereals of the Sudano-Sahelian, and maize, the roots and tubers, and tree crops are mainly cultivated in the Gulf of Guinea. With the development and release of new varieties of crops and changing climate, the distribution of these crops across ECOWAS is changing. Rice cultivation is becoming ubiquitous throughout the region as the urban population and demand for rice increase.

The production and yield of the major food and cash crops—rice, maize, millet and sorghum grains, cassava and yam tubers, groundnut (unshelled), cotton lint, coffee green berries, cocoa beans and palm oil—for the Gulf of Guinea and the Sudano-Sahelian zones are shown in **Tables 2–4**; along these lines:

3.2.1 Annual crops: cereals

The production and yield of rice in the Gulf of Guinea zone increased by 99 and 17%, respectively; for the Sudano-Sahelian zone, the corresponding values were 113 and 24%. The production of maize in the Gulf of Guinea zone rose by 53%, but yield declined by 4%. The production and yield of millet in the Gulf of Guinea zone declined by 78 and 45%, respectively. In the Sudano-Sahelian, zone production increased by 9%, but yield declined by 3%. For sorghum, production and yield in the Gulf of Guinea decreased by 31 and 14%, respectively; contrary to this, production and yield increased by 54 and 8%, respectively, in the Sudano-Sahelian zone.

3.2.2 Annual crops: roots and tubers and groundnut

The production of cassava in the Gulf of Guinea zone increased by 37%, but yield declined by 19%. In the Sudano-Sahelian zone, production and yield increased by 12 and 42%, respectively; this was a desirable case of yield increasing substantially over time. The production of yam in the Gulf of Guinea increased by 27%, but yield decreased by 25%. Similarly, the production in the Sudano-Sahelian zone increased by 157%, but yield declined by 29%. The large increase in yam production in the Sudano-Sahelian may indicate evolving farming systems because yam was traditionally a major crop in the humid areas of ECOWAS. In the Gulf of Guinea,

	Production (×1000 t)		Yield (t ha^{-1})	
	2003	2013	2003	2013
Rice (paddy)				
Gulf of Guinea	5912	11,739	1.48	1.73
Range	54.2–3116	209.7–4823	0.83–2.31	1.25–3.30
Sudano-Sahelian	1344	2863	2.35	2.91
Range	20.5–938.2	69.7–1978	1.77–3.10	1.05–6.28
ECOWAS	7256	14,602	1.59	1.88
Maize				
Gulf of Guinea	8878	13,577	1.50	1.44
Range	16–5203	7.3–8423	1.00–2.24	0.49–2.15
Sudano-Sahelian	1569	3504	1.59	1.97
Range	2.2–665.5	5.8–1636	0.38–2.28	0.18–2.59
ECOWAS	10,447	17,081	1.51	1.52
Millet				
Gulf of Guinea	6765	1474	1.32	0.72
Range	10–6260	18.1–910	0.65–1.38	0.61–1.29
Sudano-Sahelian	5938	6464	0.59	0.58
Range	120.3–2745	93.8–2922	0.48–1.09	0.41–0.94
ECOWAS	12,703	7938	0.84	0.60
Sorghum				
Gulf of Guinea	8768	6079	1.13	0.98
Range	10–8016	26.9–5300	0.55–1.16	0.67–1.35
Sudano-Sahelian	3115	4792	0.65	0.70
Range	30.1–1610	30.4–1880	0.27–1.13	0.37–1.11
ECOWAS	11,883	10,871	0.95	0.83

Source: [11, 13].

Table 2.
Cereal production in ECOWAS.

production and yield of groundnut declined by 10 and 28%, respectively. In the Sudano-Sahelian, production and yield increased by 50 and 1%, respectively.

3.2.3 Zonal effects on crop production and yield

Crop production was higher in the Gulf of Guinea than the Sudano-Sahelian zone, with Nigeria being the highest producer in ECOWAS of rice, maize, sorghum, cassava, yam, and groundnut in both 2003 and 2013. World Bank [20] also reported higher crop production in the humid and subhumid AEZs than the semiarid zone. The greater proportion of the humid and subhumid zones is within the Gulf of Guinea zone, and this may explain in part why production of the major crops was higher in this zone. The average yield of rice, maize, and yam in the Sudano-Sahelian zone was, however, higher than the average yield of these crops in the Gulf of Guinea zone in both years. Thus, the highest yield of rice in 2003 and 2013 was reported for Niger, and that of maize in 2003 was for Senegal, and in 2013 it was

	Production (×1000 t)		Yield (t ha^{-1})	
	2003	**2013**	**2003**	**2013**
Cassava				
Gulf of Guinea	55,647	76,215	10.28	8.37
Range	38–36,304	23–47,407	5.86–15.2	3.52–18.27
Sudano-Sahelian	344	384	6.86	9.75
Range	3.4–181.7	4.1–156.1	2.17–17.90	1.36–19.97
ECOWAS	55,991	76,599	10.25	8.37
Yam				
Gulf of Guinea	41,017	52,197	10.45	7.83
Range	20.5–29,697	21.5–35,618	8.67–12.11	6.61–16.78
Sudano-Sahelian	67	171	12.36	8.77
Range	31–35	79.2–91.6	12.01–12.80	5.86–20.63
ECOWAS	41,084	52,368	10.45	7.83
Groundnut				
Gulf of Guinea	4056	3664	1.34	0.97
Range	4.3–3037	6.5–2475	0.60–1.53	0.64–1.24
Sudano-Sahelian	1316	1979	0.77	0.78
Range	92.9–440.7	0.28–677.5	049–0.89	0.49–1.38
ECOWAS	5372	5643	1.13	0.89

Source: *[11, 13].*

Table 3.
Cassava, yam, and groundnut production in ECOWAS.

for Mali. In both years, the highest yield of cassava was reported for Niger and that of yam in both years for Mali. These findings are relevant in exploring how climate change may impact production and productivity differently, in various parts of ECOWAS, and how this knowledge can be exploited for improved food security and poverty alleviation.

3.2.4 Changes in crop production and yield over time

The production of rice, maize, cassava, yam, and groundnut increased between 2003 and 2013, but that of millet and sorghum decreased. In contrast to this positive change in production, yields of millet, sorghum, cassava, yam, and groundnut decreased, and although those of rice and maize increased slightly in ECOWAS as a whole, yields were low and well below their potentials. Increases in crop production in ECOWAS are generally more closely related to the area harvested than to yield per unit area [22]. Lipton et al. [23] reported yields of 1.01 t ha^{-1} for rice, 0.78 t ha^{-1} for maize, 0.56 t ha^{-1} for millet, 0.76 t ha^{-1} for sorghum, and 7.63 t ha^{-1} for cassava in Western Africa for 1961–1963. These levels, compared to those shown in **Tables** 2 and 3, indicate only modest increases over four to five decades from a very low baseline. Thus, the evidence is that while crop production increased, the boosting of crop yields (productivity), a major concern of CAADP and the Maputo Accord did not take place during the period under review. This finding should be of serious concern given that the Consultative Group on International Agricultural

	Production (×1000 t)		Yield (t ha^{-1})	
	2003	**2013**	**2003**	**2013**
Coffee green				
Gulf of Guinea	192.3	172.6	0.37	0.21
Range	0.06–140.0	0.07–103.7	0.2–1.7	0.14–2.48
Sudano-Sahelian		0.062		0.21
ECOWAS	192.3	172.7		0.76
Cocoa beans				
Gulf of Guinea	2263	2696	0.49	0.48
Range	0.1–1352	0.12–1449	0.17–0.68	0.14–0.86
ECOWAS	2263	2696	0.49	0.48
Cotton lint				
Gulf of Guinea	573	368		
Range	1.8–172	1.4–133.5		
Sudano-Sahelian	447	422		
Range	0.18–259.7	0.19–280		
ECOWAS	1020	790		
Palm oil				
Gulf of Guinea	1528	1638		
Range	4.9–1022	6–880		
Sudano-Sahelian	9	17		
Range	2.5–6	3–13.7		
ECOWAS	1537	1655		

Source: *authors calculations from [11, 13].*

Table 4.
Perennial and cash crop production in ECOWAS.

Research (CGIAR) centers in collaboration with the National Agricultural Research and Extension Systems (NARES) have developed and released high-yielding, pest- and disease-resistant crop varieties with associated improved crop and soil management practices over the past three to four decades and increase in crop yields is recognized as a major step toward poverty reduction and food security [23]. The impacts of climate change on agriculture have reinforced the need for achievement and maintenance of high crop yields as an adaptation measure both by small-scale and large-scale investors.

3.3 Perennial and cash crops

Data for coffee, cocoa, and palm oil (from oil palm) were available almost exclusively for the Gulf of Guinea zone where they are mainly cultivated. For coffee, in the Gulf of Guinea zone, production and yield decreased by 10 and 45%, respectively. Production of cocoa increased by 19%, while yield decreased by 3%. Cote d'Ivoire in 2003 and 2013 was the highest producer in ECOWAS of coffee green berries and cocoa beans. Like for annual crops, yields of cocoa and coffee were well below potentials, and their improvement should be a sector development priority for governments. Production of palm oil increased by 7% in the Gulf of Guinea and 96% in the Sudano-Sahelian zone (data only for Gambia and Senegal), but the production of cotton lint in the Gulf of Guinea and Sudano-Sahelian zone declined by 36 and 6%, respectively. This contrasts with the 7.3% per annum increase in cotton production between 1980 and 2006 in West Africa reported by [21]. Mali in 2003 and Burkina Faso in 2013 were the highest producers of cotton lint in ECOWAS. Data were not available on yield of palm oil and cotton.

4. Economic factors: GDP, inflation, infrastructure, and trade

The vulnerability of the ECOWAS agricultural system to climate change depends partly on certain economic factors such as income, price level, labor productivity, transportation, communication, innovation, and trade, which define ECOWAS' adaptive capacity to external shocks, including climate change. The greater the adaptive capacity of ECOWAS, the lower its vulnerability to climate change, particularly in the agricultural sector.

4.1 Growth, inflation, and capital formation

After several years of strong economic growth, ECOWAS faced a small increase in 2016 of 0.5%. It rebounded in 2017 to 2.5% and was projected to 3.8% in 2018 and 3.9% in 2019. Countries' performance varied, but because Nigeria, Cote d'Ivoire, Ghana, and Senegal contribute to about 90% of the regional gross domestic product (GDP), their patterns largely shape regional ones. In 2003, agriculture was the dominant sector in ECOWAS (about 40% of GDP), but services contributed most to GDP in Liberia and Sierra Leone soon after the end of their civil wars which devastated the agriculture sector; however, agriculture remains dominant in 2013 [24].

GDP per capita increased by 31.3% in ECOWAS, 34.8% in the Gulf of Guinea, and 26.9% in Sudano-Sahelian between 2003 and 2013 (**Table 5**), indicating an increase in standard of living. Furthermore, consumer prices almost double during the same period, threatening the positive effect of the increased income. Changes in the productive capacity of ECOWAS captured by the gross capital formation represented a larger share of the GDP in 2013 than 2003. The same trend is observed in the Gulf of Guinea and Sudano-Sahelian zones. Agricultural labor productivity increased by 22% between 2003 and 2013 in ECOWAS, while it decreased by 18% in Sudano-Sahelian zone. This may be explained partly by an increase in fertilizer consumption in ECOWAS and in both agroecological zones (**Table 5**).

Financing adaptation and mitigation are an important component of building resilient of the agricultural sector to climate change in ECOWAS. As observed in the previous paragraph, increasing income per capita, investment, and labor productivity are an indication that further economic efficiency in production may be realized in ECOWAS to support the financing of mitigation and adaptation efforts for climate change. However, higher consumer prices represent a significant challenge that may offset the positive effect of an improved efficiency in production for climate finance. Furthermore climate change compounds with other pressing socioeconomic development challenges such as education, sanitation, health and infrastructure, resulting to underinvestment in agriculture in ECOWAS. As reported by AfDB [25], the agriculture sector in ECOWAS suffers from chronic underinvestment. Only Burkina Faso, Mali, Niger, and Senegal have so far raised public expenditure to 10% of GDP, the target fixed by the Maputo Declaration in 2003. The Gambia, Ghana, and Togo are on the threshold of reaching this target. Nigeria devotes 6% of GDP to agriculture and the remaining ECOWAS countries

Zone/ region	GDP per capita (constant 2010 US$)		Consumer price index (2010 = 100)		Gross capital formation (percentage of GDP)		Agriculture, value added per worker (constant 2010 US$)		Fertilizer consumption (kilograms per hectare of arable land)	
	2003	2013	2003	2013	2003	2013	2003	2013	2003	2013
Gulf of Guinea										
Total					144.3	165.2				
Mean	736.0	992.1	64.7	122.5	9.1–23.8	7.2–27.8	1030.9	1584.7	8.6	16.3
Range	271.0–1426.9	383.1–2475.9	40.8–83.6	108.2–156.4			420.0–2445.3	521.5–5041.1	0.8–29.3	2.9–37.2
Sudano-Sahelian										
Total					90.2	165.5				
Mean	870.1	1104.0	80.7	108.4			1215.3	996.9	7.8	12.1
Range	335.7–2310.5	373.7–3389.9	67.7–85.2	105.6–115.5	10.0–22.3	17.8–36.2	544.7–1960.8	470.5–1298.5	0.3–10.9	0.4–31.5
ECOWAS	789.6	1036.9	72.1	116.9	234.5	330.7	1107.7	1349.6	8.2	14.4

Source: *Authors calculations from the World Bank Open Data [23].*

Table 5.
Growth, inflation, and capital formation.

less than 5%. This is not surprising because in the presence of limited resources and a range of objectives, financing agricultural development issues such as climate change should involve trade-offs among multiple policy goals. Therefore, financing climate policies, programs, and plans in the agricultural sector of ECOWAS should be prioritized not only in terms of their ability to reduce the impact of climate change but also in terms of their ability to deliver some development outcomes.

4.2 Infrastructure development

Infrastructure development in ECOWAS can be analyzed in three key areas: communication, transport, and technology. The telecommunication priority is the development of a reliable and modern regional telecom broadband infrastructure including the INTELCOM II program, alternative broadband infrastructure, and submarine cables as well as the establishment of a single liberalized telecom market. By 2013, 11 coastal member states were connected to submarine cables with at least 1 new landing station, and the 3 landlocked countries (Burkina Faso, Mali, and Niger) now have at least 2 access routes to the submarine cables. This has substantially increased the percentage of people using the Internet (from 1.1% in 2003 to 9.9% in 2013) and number of subscriptions to mobile cellular (from 4 subscriptions in 2003 to 78.4 subscriptions in 2013 per 100 people). A similar trend is observed in Gulf of Guinea and Sudano-Sahelian zones.

The transport program in ECOWAS has overseen the implementation of multimodal transport infrastructure and policies to promote physical cohesion among member states and to facilitate the movement of persons, goods, and services within the community with special emphasis on increased access to island and landlocked countries. However, the transportation infrastructure is still underdeveloped and of poor quality. For example, the quality of port infrastructure was estimated at 3.9 on a scale of 7, the latter representing a well-developed and efficient infrastructure by international standards. Rail lines decreased by 72% between 2003 and 2013. This is mainly due to a sharp decrease of rail lines in the Gulf of Guinea zone (**Table 6**).

ECOWAS countries still have a long way to go to reach the African Union's target of devoting 1% of GDP to gross domestic expenditure on research and development (GERD). Mali comes closest (0.66% in 2010), followed by Senegal (0.54% in 2010), according to the UNESCO Science Report [25]. There is a lack of researchers in ECOWAS in general. AfDB [25] highlighted that only Senegal stands out, with 361 full-time equivalent (FTE) researchers per million population in 2010, while other countries, where data was available, have less than 60. However, the number of trademark applications, as an indicator of innovation, has increased substantially between 2003 and 2013 from 1671 to 25,294. Almost all trademark applications are from the Gulf of Guinea zone (99%).

Infrastructure development is an important means to build resilience to climate change, particularly in the agricultural sector, because it also delivers vital development outcomes. We should recognize that the availability and quality of infrastructure are never substitutes to agriculture-specific policies such as an increase in fertilizer use, irrigation, and improved seeds. However, inadequate infrastructure may be a significant constraint to growth and productivity. Indeed, recent literature indicates a significant positive link between infrastructure and agricultural productivity [26]. For example, transport infrastructure provides important connectivity with growing markets and also reduces input costs and transaction costs for producers and consumers, particularly in the context of climate change. Furthermore, information acquisition costs can represent a significant obstacle, for instance, when climate and weather data are costly or difficult to access. Improvement in communication infrastructure represents an opportunity to reduce information acquisition costs, thereby strengthening farmers' responses to external shocks such as climate change.

Zone/Region	Individuals using the Internet (percentage of the population)		Mobile cellular subscriptions (per 100 people)		Trademark applications, total		Quality of port infrastructure, WEF[a]		Rail lines (total route-km)	
	2003	2013	2003	2013	2003	2013	2003	2013	2003	2013
Gulf of Guinea										
Total					1313.0	24,888.0			4482.0	639.0
Mean	0.7	7.8	2.9	73.7			0.0	3.7		
Range	0.0–1.4	3.1–19.1	0.1–7.2	55.9–106.4	627–686.0	14–19332.0	0.0–0.0	3.2–4.5	977–3505.0	639–639.0
Sodano-Sahelian										
Total					358.0	406.0			0	622.0
Mean	1.6	13.1	5.8	85.4			0.0	4.1		
Range	0.2–4.3	1.15–37.5	0.7–11.6	38.0–119.9	25–298.0	406.0–406.0	0.0–0.0	3.5–4.8	0.0–0.0	622.0–622.0
ECOWAS	1.1	9.9	4.0	78.4	1671.0	25,294.0	0.0	3.9	4482.0	1261.0

a: 1, extremely underdeveloped, to 7, well developed and efficient by international standards).
***Source:** Authors' calculations from the World Bank Open Data [23].*

Table 6.
Infrastructure development.

Recent literature also recognizes that innovation (technological, managerial, and institutional) in agriculture is clearly an important response for effective and equitable adaptation to and mitigation of climate change. As underlined by Llanto [27], innovation can enhance technology adoption, may prevent or facilitate migration of production/population, enhance trade and aid, and increase efficiency of insurance and feasibility of inventories. More importantly, innovation will be the key in moving toward climate-smart agriculture.

4.3 Trade development

ECOWAS has a huge potential for trade both in global and intra-regional terms mainly because of its large natural resource endowment, agricultural potential, and intra-regional complementarities. Trade (the sum of exports and imports of goods and services) was estimated at almost 65% of GDP in 2003 and 78% of the GDP in 2013, representing an increase of 13 points in 10 years. A similar trend is observed in Gulf of Guinea and Sudano-Sahelian zones. The export profile of ECOWAS shows little product diversity, with a heavy reliance on extractive products (e.g., petroleum, natural gas) and a few agricultural commodities (e.g., cocoa, rubber, cotton). Agricultural raw material exports measured as a share of merchandise exports decreased by 12 points between 2003 and 2013. The decrease is substantial in Sudano-Sahelian zone (20 points) and moderate in the Gulf of Guinea zone (5 points). However, food exports measured as a share of merchandise exports increased by 19 points in the Sudano-Sahelian zone and decreased by 15 points in the Gulf of Guinea zone (**Table 7**). This is an indication of an improvement in the industrialization of ECOWAS and/or building of adaptive capacity to environmental and economic shocks, such as climate change.

ECOWAS imports are more diversified, with a high share of industrialized products (e.g., refined petroleum, vehicles, ships, telecommunication equipment)

Zone/ region	Trade (percentage of GDP)		Agricultural raw material imports (percentage of merchandise imports)		Agricultural raw material exports (percentage of merchandise exports)		Food imports (percentage of merchandise imports)		Food exports (percentage of merchandise exports)	
	2003	2013	2003	2013	2003	2013	2003	2013	2003	2013
Gulf of Guinea										
Total										
Mean	67.9	81.1	1.3	1.3	17.9	13.1	26.3	20.9	37.4	22.9
Range	43.3–102.5	31.0–131.0	0.4–4.0	0.4–2.8	0.0–74.2	3.2–49.1	15.5–62.4	14.2–40.3	0.0–95.4	4.9–38.5
Sudano-Sahelian										
Total										
Mean	60.4	72.9	2.0	1.3	29.4	9.8	28.1	27.7	32.5	51.3
Range	30.7–98.8	61.7–95.3	0.7–4.3	0.4–2.6	3.3–79.5	0.0–44.4	18.0–37.6	12.1–37.3	6.4–85.9	8.0–92.0
ECOWAS	64.9	77.8	1.7	1.3	23.6	11.6	27.2	24.0	34.9	35.8

***Source:** authors calculations from the World Bank Open Data [23].*

Table 7.
Trade development.

and food products (e.g., rice, wheat). Agricultural raw material imports measured as a share of merchandise imports decreased slightly by 0.4 points between 2003 and 2013. The same trend is observed in Sudano-Sahelian and Gulf of Guinea zones. On the other hand, food imports measured as a share of merchandise imports decreased in ECOWAS (3.2 points), Sudano-Sahelian zone (0.4 points), and Gulf of Guinea zone (5.4 points) between 2003 and 2013. ECOWAS main trading partners are highly industrialized countries such as China, India, the USA, EU countries, and Brazil, which mainly buy raw materials and sell industrialized products from/to the region. Intra-regional trade takes place, but is mainly, unreported, informal and generally considered to be well below its potential [29].

Trade is crucial for economic growth and food security, thereby representing an important controlling factor for climate change impacts in the agricultural sector [28]. Torres and van Seters [29] showed that while some countries in ECOWAS may be experiencing good crop harvest, others may not due to stochastic patterns in climate. The authors demonstrated that acreage and crop production in ECOWAS countries are sensitive to climate change and climate change will lead to a shift in land use for agricultural production within and among countries as a rational response to its impact on crop yield by farmers seeking to maximize the profit of their farm activities. A structural transformation of the agricultural sector is, therefore, inevitable to offset the negative impacts of climate change to achieve a better level of livelihood for the population. This means, therefore, that one of the ways to resolve the issue of food availability may be through food trade across countries. Several arguments have been made in favor of trade of agricultural commodities as a means of adapting to climate change [30, 31]. First, trade operates as an insurance against the risk of climate change. Going by this view, trade is the means by which food availability can be preserved for regions that are affected by reduced agricultural productivity. Second, trade can spread the cost of adaptation if free trade flows are allowed. In fact, if free trade is allowed between countries, countries that are net exporters of food may face food price increase in order to allow other food-deficit regions to survive.

5. Economics of adaptation to climate change in the agriculture sector

Recent literature on the impact of future climate change on West African crop yields showed a large dispersion of yield changes ranging from −50 to +90%, with the median yield loss near −11% [32]. The predicted impact is larger in Sudano-Sahelian region (−18% median response) than in the Gulf of Guinea (−13%). Roudier et al. [32] highlighted that the consistently negative impact of climate change results mainly from the temperature whose increase projected by climate models is much larger relative to precipitation change. As discussed in previous sections, the vulnerability of the biophysical system and the underdeveloped economic system of ECOWAS will exacerbate this impact on agriculture and food security. Economic analysis of adaptation in the agriculture sector of ECOWAS is still in its infancy state, and information even on costs benefit analysis of adaptation options in the agriculture sector of ECOWAS is scarce. Nevertheless, some valuable information on the magnitudes of costs and returns on a country-wide and technology-specific basis has emerged.

Butt et al. [33], through modeling studies, showed that for Mali, policy changes that result in reduction in soil productivity loss, cropland expansion, adoption of improved cultivars, and changes in trade patterns altogether, under climate change, showed an annual gain of $252 million in economic benefits as opposed to a $161 million loss without policy adjustment. Roudier et al. [32] examined the benefits of climate change adaptation in agriculture for Ghana when the whole adaptation resource envelope is spent on gradual expansion of irrigated land area from 2012 onwards. The assumed upfront investment cost of irrigation is $18,000 per ha, taking account of Ghana-specific cost estimates for recent and planned irrigation projects plus the need for complementary investment in water harvesting, etc. Under the general circulation model (GCM)/Special Report on Emissions Scenarios (SRES) of the IPCC modeling global wet scenario, the share of irrigated land rises gradually from less than 0.4 to 15% of the current total cultivated area. The resulting average annual factor productivity increase for agriculture as a whole is an additional 0.36% above baseline productivity growth. They also pointed out that this scenario can also be interpreted as representing other productivity-rising agricultural adaptation measures with a comparable yield impact per dollar spent.

It is well known that technological adaptations such as adoption of high-yielding pest and disease-resistant varieties of climate-smart varieties of cassava can double crop yields even without the use of expensive inputs (and therefore positive returns), in the immediate term. On the other hand, adaptation options in the form of soil conservation practices such as contour ridges and agroforestry require investments to pay off over longer periods, which small-scale farmers cannot afford in the typical situation of lack of long-term credit facilities by commercial banks. Persons with precarious hold on the land, such as women and strangers, are particularly constrained to make such investments. Thus, World Bank [34] reported that while farmers in Nigeria who were dependent on leased and/or communal lands expressed implicit dislike for climate-smart agriculture (CSA)-related investments, the majority with freehold titles, particularly those with registered titles, expressed positive willingness-to-accept incentives to embrace CSA and combat land degradation [35].

The following examples illustrate the nature of the investments and returns in soil management adaptation options in ECOWAS: in the Sahel of ECOWAS, stone bunds associated with shallow pits, filled with compost or manure (Zai pits), requiring 30–50 t of stones ha^{-1} and costing \$200 ha^{-1} and 150 person days of labor ha^{-1} for constructing the bunds on contours, have resulted in doubling of millet yields [36]. Bjorkemar [37] estimated the potential returns over 25 years from agroforestry, in a village in the Bombali District of Sierra Leone, as follows: $15,470, $135,812, $5,427,800, and $11,903,090 for dispersed interplanting, boundary planting, and woodlot and fruit orchard, respectively. A World Agroforestry Center study reported by [36] showed that farmer-managed natural regeneration raised millet yields from 150 to 500 kg ha^{-1} in Maradi, Niger, taking into consideration improvement in soil fertility, and increased supply of food, fodder, and firewood was at least a \$56 ha^{-1} return each year.

Analysis of the economics of adaptation to climate change is moving from a focus on efficiency, market solutions, and cost-benefit analysis of adaptation to include "multi-metric" considerations of non-monetary and nonmarket measures, risks, inequities, and behavioral biases and barriers and limits and consideration of ancillary benefits and costs for providing support to decision-makers [31]. An understanding of the controlling factors of climate change impact chain is useful as inputs to these kinds of analysis. A few studies on economics of adaptation to climate change in ECOWAS have reached such sophistication. Recently, Aklesso et al. [38] tried to integrate a number of biophysical and economic factors of climate change impact chain in order to analyze the potential of intra-regional trade in ECOWAS for increasing food availability in the context of climate change. Several models were integrated: a regional climate model to predict temperature and precipitations from 2004 to 2100 with two representative concentration pathways (RCPs); an econometric crop simulator to simulate crop yield under RCPs; a bioeconomic optimization model to predict agricultural land allocation and crop production under RCPs; and an intra-regional food trade module built from a classical transportation model to allocate food optimally from excess supply countries to excess demand countries. The authors showed that the climate-induced trade pattern in ECOWAS depends on the prevailing socioeconomic conditions during the century, and several countries may become dependent on food imports outside ECOWAS. However, doubling crop yields by 2050 and adjusting the ECOWAS common external tariffs could significantly reduce outside dependence. Although this study attempts to investigate the link between climate change and food security in ECOWAS, more research is needed to understand how the integration of factors of climate change impact chain could affect food security and promote sustainable agricultural development in ECOWAS.

6. Conclusion

This chapter assessed key biophysical and economic factors of the climate change impact chain and the economics of adaptation in the agricultural sector of ECOWAS.

As in many developing regions, land for agricultural production in ECOWAS has increased at the expense of forest land. These changes vary, however, by agroecological zones. Furthermore, ECOWAS countries have experienced significant land degradation. The primary causes of land degradation are deforestation, agriculture, conversion of grasslands to croplands, and overgrazing. Cropping systems are generally related to agroecological zones; however, the release of new varieties of crops and changing climate is significantly changing the distribution of crops across ECOWAS. Crop production was higher in the Gulf of Guinea than the Sudano-Sahelian zone. This is partly explained by the high proportion of humid and sub-humid zones within the Gulf of Guinea. Increases in crop production in ECOWAS are more often related to the area harvested than to yield per unit area, which is the major concern of CAADP and the Maputo Accord. The boost in crop productivity expected from CAADP and the Maputo Accord did not happen between 2003 and 2013. Increasing crop yields through agricultural intensification while reducing land degradation is critical to reduce the impact of climate change in the agricultural sector of ECOWAS.

In recent years, ECOWAS has experienced an increase in income per capita, investment, and labor productivity, indicating that further economic efficiency in production may be realized. This may boost climate financing in the agricultural sector. However, further improvement in general production may not generate enough resources to address both climate change and other development challenges, particularly in the context of increasing prices. There is a need for policy makers to prioritize climate strategies that also have some development impacts. Infrastructure in ECOWAS is underdeveloped with poor quality. Although the availability and quality of infrastructure may never substitute for agriculture-specific policies such as an increase fertilizer use, irrigation, and improved seeds, infrastructure development can help build resilience to climate change. Indeed, infrastructure development provides important connectivity with growing markets and also reduces input, transaction, and information acquisition costs for farmers and other actors in the agricultural sector of ECOWAS. On the other hand, ECOWAS has a huge potential for trade both in global and intra-regional terms mainly because of its large natural resource endowment, agricultural potential, and intra-regional complementarities. However, intra-regional trade that takes place in ECOWAS is mainly informal and generally considered to be well below its potential.

In the context of insufficient financial resources to support climate adaptation actions, stimulating trade appears as an appropriate measure to preserve food availability by allowing countries with excess food production to trade with food-deficit countries.

Returns to adaptation to climate change in ECOWAS can vary widely depending on the technology with gains of up to $252 million in economic benefits compared to $161 loss without policy adjustment in a country in the Sudano-Sahelian zone. The economics of adaptation to climate change in the agricultural sector of ECOWAS has focused so far on the magnitude of costs and returns on a country-wide and technology-specific measures. There is a need, however, for further research to integrate biophysical and economic factors of climate change impact chain in sound analytical frameworks to provide "multi-metric" considerations of non-monetary and nonmarket measures, risks, inequities, and behavioral biases in addressing climate change.

Although important results were obtained regarding the biophysical and economic opportunities and challenges for building the resilience of the agriculture sector of ECOWAS to climate change, our study presents some limitations. For example, a detailed year-to-year trend analysis from 2003 to 2013 is not done because of the wide scope of the study (mapping), and data are not available for some parameters for some countries, and some data are not available for the same years for all variables studied. In addition, the environmental and social factors that are not covered in the study are equally important in defining the climate change impact chain in the agricultural sectors. These issues will be addressed in further research.

Author details

Calvin Atewamba[1]* and Edward R. Rhodes[2]

1 United Nations University Institute for Natural Resources in Africa, Toronto, Canada

2 Njala University, PMB, Freetown, Sierra Leone

*Address all correspondence to: atewamba@gmail.com

References

[1] FAO. Irrigation in Africa: AQUASTAT Survey. Rome: Food and Agriculture Organization of the United Nations; 2005

[2] UNCDP. List of Least Developed Countries. New York: United Nations Committee for Development Policy; 2016

[3] FAO. Agroecological Map of West Africa. FAO; 2016 [Online]. Available from: www.fao.org/docrep/006/y4751e/y4751e0p.htm [Accessed: 17-10-2018]

[4] Maplecroft. Climate change vulnerability index 2014. Maplecroft; 2013 [Online]. Available from: https://reliefweb.int/sites/reliefweb.int/files/resources/Climate_Change_Vulnerability_Index_%202014_Map_0.pdf [Accessed: 12-12-2016]

[5] Kurukulasuriya P, Mendelsohn R. How Will Climate Change Shift Agroecological Zones and Impact African Agriculture? Policy Research Working Paper 4717. Washington: World Bank; 2008

[6] Nelson GC, Rosegrant M, Koo J, Robertson R, Sulser T, Zhu T, et al. Climate Change: Impact on Agriculture and Costs of Adaptation. Washington: International Food Policy Research Institute; 2009

[7] Jalloh A, Nelson G, Thomas T, Zougmore R, Roy-Macauley H. West African Agriculture and Climate Change. Washington: International Food Policy Research Institute; 2013

[8] Rhodes E, Jalloh A, Diouf A. Review of Research and Policies for Climate Change Adaptation in the Agriculture Sector in West Africa. Brighton: AfricaInteract, Institute of Development Studies; 2014

[9] Roudier P, Ducharne A, Feyen L. Climate change impacts on run off in West Africa: A review. Hydrology and Earth System Sciences. 2014;**18**:2789-2801

[10] World Bank. World Development Indicators. Washington: International Bank for Reconstruction and Development; 2005

[11] Rhodes ER, Atewamba C. Climate change impact chain factors in ECOWAS. Journal of Agriculture and Environment for International Development. 2019;**113**(1):35-78

[12] FAO. Land Use. FAO; 2018 [Online]. Available: www.fao.org/statistics/en [Accessed: 15-09-2018]

[13] FAO. Agricultural Production Data. 2018 [Online]. Available: www.fao.org/statistics/en [Accessed: 15-09-2018]

[14] World Bank. World Development Indicators. Washington: International Bank for Reconstruction and Development; 2015

[15] Le Q, Nkonya E, Mirzabaev A. Biomass Productivity-Based Mapping of Global Level Degradation Hotspots. Bonn: ZEF, University of Bonn; 2014

[16] Kaufman JB, Bhomia R. Ecosystem carbon stocks of mangroves across broad environmental gradients in west-Central Africa: Global and regional comparisons. PLoS One. 2017;**12**(11)

[17] Bot A, Nachtergale F, Young A. Land resource potential and constraints at regional and country levels. In: World Soil Resources Report 90. Food and Agriculture Organization of the United Nations: Rome; 2000

[18] Nkonya E, Johnson T, Kwon H, Kato E. Economics of land degradation in Sub-Saharan Africa. In: Economics of Land Degradation and Improvement—A Global Assessment for

Sustainable Development. Washington & Bonn: International Food Policy Research Institute & Center for Development Research (ZEF); 2016

[19] Moussa B, Nkonya E, Meyer S, Kato S, Johnson T, Hawking J. Economics of land degradation in Niger. In: Economics of Land Degradation and Improvement: A Global Assessment for Sustainable Development. Washington & Bonn: International Food Policy Research Institute & Center for Development Research (ZEF), University of Bonn; 2016

[20] World Bank. Africa's Development in a Changing Climate. Washington: International Bank for Reconstruction and Development; 2009

[21] Blein R, Soule B, Dupraigre B, Yerima B. Agricultural Potential of West Africa (ECOWAS). Presles: Fondation Pour l'agriculture et la Ruralité Dans le Monde; 2008

[22] Rhodes E, Tambi E, Bangali S. State of knowledge on CSA in Africa: Case studies from Burkina Faso, Senegal, and Sierra Leone. In: Forum for Agricultural Research in Africa, Accra. 2015

[23] Lipton M. Learning from Others: Increasing Agricultural Productivity for Human Development. Washington, USA: United Nations Development Programme; 2012

[24] World Bank. World Bank Open Data. The World Bank; 2018 [Online]. Available: https://data.worldbank.org/indicator [Accessed: 1-12-2018]

[25] AfDB. West Africa Economic Outlook West Africa Economic Outlook. Abidjan, Côte d'Ivoire: AfDB; 2018

[26] UNESCO. UNESCO Science Report: Towards 2030. Paris, France: United Nations Educational, Scientific and Cultural Organization; 2015

[27] Llanto GM. The impact of infrastructure on agricultural productivity. Journal of Developing Areas. 2012;**28**(4):469-486

[28] Zilberman D, Lipper L, McCarthy N, Gordon B. Innovation in response to climate change. In: Climate Smart Agriculture: Building Resilience to Climate Change. Vol. 52. Springer; 2018

[29] Torres C, van Seters J. Overview of Trade and Barriers to Trade in West Africa: Insights in Political Economy Dynamics, with Particular Focus on Agricultural and Food Trade. Maastricht: European Center for Development Policy Management; 2016

[30] Lokonon BK, Egbendewe AYG, Atewamba C. Spatial Implications of Climate Change on Land Allocation and Agricultural Production in ECOWAS. Vol. 17. Accra, Accra, Ghana: United Nations University Institute for Natural Resources in Africa; 2016

[31] Stephan G, Schenker O. International Trade and the Adaptation to Climate Change and Variability. Mannheim, Germany: ZEW - Center for European Economic Research; 2012

[32] Roudier P, Sultan B, Quirion P, Berg A. The impact of future climate change on West African crop yields: What does the recent literature say? Global Environmental Change. 2011;**21**(3):1073-1083

[33] Butt T, McCarl B, Kergna A. Policies for reducing agricultural vulnerability to climate change in Mali. Climate Policy. 2006;**5**:583-598

[34] World Bank. The Economics of Adaptation to Climate Change: A Synthesis Report. Washington: International Bank for Reconstruction and Development; 2010

[35] Shittu A, Kehinde M, Ogunnaike M, Oyawole F. Effects of land tenure and

property rights on farm households' willingness to accept incentives to invest in measures to combat land degradation in Nigeria. Agricultural and Resource Economics Review. 2018;**47**(2):357-387

[36] Neate P. Water harvesting boosts yield in the Sahel. In: Climate Smart Agriculture Success Stories from Farming Communities Around the World. CGIAR Research Programme on Climate Change, Agriculture and Food Security (CCAFS) and Technical Center for Agriculture for Agricultural and Rural Cooperation (CTA); 2013

[37] Bjorkemar K. Agroforestry in Sierra Leone: Examining the Economic Potential with Carbon Sequestration. Sweden: Linnaeus University; 2014

[38] Aklesso YGE, Lokonon BOK, Atewemba C, Coulibaly N. Can intra-regional food trade increase food availability in the context of global climatic change in West Africa? Climatic Change. 2017;**145**(1-2):101

Chapter 6

Mercury Cycling in the Gulf of Gdańsk (Southern Baltic Sea)

Dominika Saniewska

Abstract

The most efficient way of mercury (Hg) transport to the Gulf of Gdańsk was river runoff. Therefore, hydrological conditions were the most important factors controlling the inflow of Hg to the sea. The second most important Hg source in the Gulf was atmospheric deposition, which transported seven times smaller load than rivers. The Hg wet deposition dominated in the warm season, while during the heating season the predominant was dry deposition of mercury. The Hg source, which should not be neglected during the creation of the mass balance of Hg in aquatic ecosystems, was the coastal erosion. In the Gulf of Gdańsk, it accounts for 6% of the Hg load reaching the sea. The main sink of Hg was bottom sediments. Other important processes that reduced the Hg load in the Gulf water were re-emission of Hg to the atmosphere and export of this metal to the Baltic Proper. The mass balance of mercury in the Gulf of Gdańsk indicated that a larger load of this metal flowed into the Gulf than left it. Consequently, the Gulf of Gdańsk should be treated as a cleansing zone for the Baltic Proper.

Keywords: mass balance, sea, river, atmosphere, sediments, organisms

1. Introduction

Mercury (Hg) is considered to be one of the most toxic metals found in terrestrial and aquatic ecosystems around the world. This is due to the specific nature of this element—volatility, persistence, and strong toxicity of its organic forms. It has no known essential biological function. Hg is toxic in every form; however, its toxicity depends mainly on its chemical form. The most dangerous form of Hg is methyl mercury (MeHg). Hg has neurotoxic, mutagenic, cytotoxic, nephrotoxic, and allergenic properties. It can also affect the functioning of the muscular system and many enzymes and proteins. Mercury is particularly dangerous for pregnant women because MeHg can easily pass through the placenta via active transport by amino acid carriers, causing embryotoxic and teratogenic effects in the fetus [1]. The aquatic environment is particularly sensitive to Hg contamination because this metal accumulates and biomagnifies with increasing trophic level [2]. Consequently, the Hg concentration in tissues of fish, birds, and water mammals can be even 100,000 times higher than in surrounding water [2]. The most common cause of Hg poisoning is consumption of predatory fish and seafood with high levels of this metal in its tissues [2]. Therefore, an understanding of mercury cycling in the aquatic environments is of fundamental importance, especially in coastal areas of densely populated countries which are usually exposed to pollutants from various human activities.

The Gulf of Gdańsk is located in the southern part of the Baltic Sea (**Figure 1**). Its northern boundary is the straight line connecting Cape Rozewie (54°50'N, 18°20'E) with Cape Taran (54°58'N, 19°59'E). The Gulf of Gdańsk (average depth 50 m, maximum depth 118 m) is often considered a separate natural region [3, 4]. Its area is 4940 km^2, while the volume of water is estimated at 291.2 km^3 [4, 5]. The hydrological conditions in the Gulf of Gdańsk are largely influenced by river inflow, of which the Vistula is the most important. It is the longest river that flows into the Baltic Sea and the second, after the Neva, in terms of the size of the catchment [6]. The Vistula catchment (194 thousand km^2) constitutes over 88% of the whole drainage basin of it of Gdańsk (220 thousand km^2) [4]. Therefore, the Gulf is considered as an important transition between land and sea. In addition, urbanized and industrialized regions within its coast affect the level of pollutants in the sea.

Investigations performed in the 1970s and 1980s revealed that the Gulf of Gdańsk was one of the most polluted water bodies in the world [7, 8]. However, the latest research indicates that the Gulf of Gdańsk is not exceptionally contaminated, and contaminant concentration in the water generally indicates a good environmental state [9]. Such considerable differences between results within the last 40 years were the effect of both analytical errors and reduction of Hg load introduced from anthropogenic sources [6]. However, this situation has caused numerous studies of environmental pollution being carried out in this area for many years, including those relating to mercury. This enabled the creation of a large database containing the results of determinations of this metal in practically all the abiotic and biotic matrices. Therefore, the objectives of this study were to construct a multi-year mass balance of Hg in the Gulf of Gdańsk. This mass balance was used to identify and better understand the dominant mercury sources and sinks in the gulf and can provide an initial basis for future research in this region.

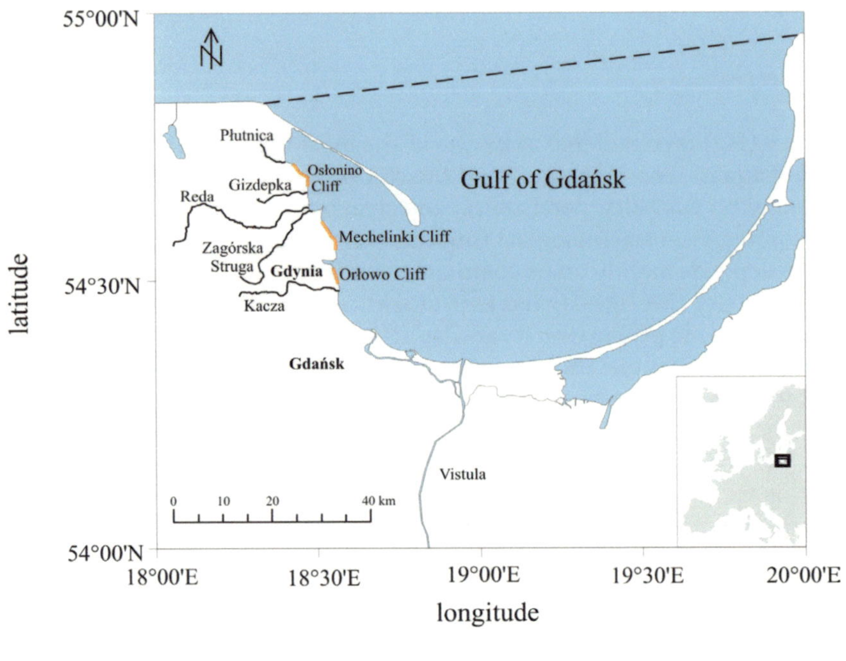

Figure 1.
The map of the study area.

2. Methods of mass balance calculations

The mass balance of mercury in the Gulf of Gdańsk was constructed on the basis of the analysis of Hg loads in precipitation, aerosols, river water, groundwater, sea water, cliff and marine sediment as well as in organism samples. In order to balance the loads of Hg in the gulf, it was assumed that the main sources of this metal were atmospheric deposition, river water, and coastal erosion, while the factors having impact on the decrease of Hg concentration in sea water were re-emission of gaseous Hg to the atmosphere, sedimentation processes, and exchange of water between the Gulf of Gdańsk and the Baltic Proper.

2.1 Sampling

Aerosols and precipitation samples were collected at a station located in Gdynia (**Figure 1**), at a distance of about 500 meters from the sea (54°30'N, 18°32'E). A detailed description of the station can be found in the publications [10, 11]. Precipitation samples were collected from August 2008 to May 2009 and from January to December 2012. In the first period, samples were collected using a bulk collector composed of a Teflon funnel of 20 cm diameter connected directly to a borosilicate glass bottle. In the second period, precipitation samples were collected using an automatic collector of wet deposition. After collection, samples were stored at −20°C until analysis. In each case, information about the amount of precipitation was obtained. Detailed information about sampling and storage methods can be found in the publications [11, 12].

Aerosol samples were collected from December 2007 to December 2008 in 24 h cycles using open-faced Teflon filter packs on 47 mm glass-fiber filters. Samples were then stored at −20°C until analysis. The collection and storage methods were described by Bełdowska et al. [10].

River water samples were taken from cross sections close to the mouth: the Vistula (12 km from mouth), the Reda (1.0 km from mouth), the Zagórska Struga (0.8 km from mouth), the Płutnica (0.4 km from mouth), the Kacza River (0.1 km from mouth), and the Gizdepka (0.6 km from mouth) (**Figure 1**). Sampling took place between 2008 and 2016 (with gaps). In each case, information about river flow was obtained. Water samples were collected directly into acid-washed borosilicate vials with Teflon screw cap. Samples were stored at 4°C until analysis. Detailed information on characteristics of the rivers as well as sampling and storage methods can be found in the publications [12–17].

The Hg concentration in groundwater was described by Szymczycha et al. [18]. The research was conducted in the Puck Bay (part of the Gulf of Gdańsk) in 2009–2010. Groundwater samples were collected directly into acid-washed borosilicate vials with Teflon screw cap and stored at 4°C until analysis. Detailed information on characteristics of the research area and sampling and storage methods can be found in the publication [18].

Information about Hg concentration in cliff deposits was presented in the work by Bełdowska et al. [12] and Kwasigroch et al. [19]. Samples were collected in two periods: 2011–2014 [12] and 2016–2017 [19]. Materials within the colluvium were collected from three cliffs located on the west part of the Gulf of Gdańsk (Orłowo, Mechelinki and Osłonino cliffs) (**Figure 1**). Detailed information about sampling and storage methods can be found in the publications [12, 19].

Seawater samples were collected between 2006 and 2016 (with gaps) [14, 15, 20–22]. As part of these studies, samples were taken from various regions of the Gulf of Gdańsk (coastal and offshore areas) as well as from different depths (surface water and profiles). Water samples were collected directly into acid-washed borosilicate vials with Teflon screw cap. Samples were stored at 4°C until analysis. Detailed information on characteristics of the stations as well as sampling and storage methods can be found in the publications [14, 15, 20–22].

The Hg concentration in sediments from several areas of the southern Baltic Sea was described by Bełdowski et al. [23], Jędruch et al. [24], and Kwasigroch et al. [19]. Samples were collected in the periods 1999–2002 [23], 2011–2013 [24], and 2016–2017 [19]. Detailed information about sampling and storage methods can be found in the publications [19, 23, 24].

Information about Hg in marine organisms was obtained from the literature [25–33]. The Hg concentration in phytoplankton was measured by Bełdowska and Kobos between 2011 and 2013 [25, 26]. Phytoplankton samples were collected with 20 μm nets and then stored at −20°C until analysis. At the same time, zooplankton samples were collected by Bełdowska and Mudrak-Cegiołak [27]. The samples were collected vertically using a zooplankton net (mesh size 50 μm). The collected samples were transported to the laboratory in life-supporting conditions and after about 24 h (required for the acclimatization and defecation of the zooplankton) live zooplankton was separated from other material using the phototaxis phenomenon. Samples were then stored at −20°C until analysis. Detailed information about sampling and storage methods can be found in the publications [25–27].

The Hg concentration in macrophytobenthos was described by Bełdowska et al. [28]. Benthic plant samples were collected along the Gulf of Gdańsk coastal zone in the years 2006–2012. The collected material was taken to the laboratory, cleansed of epiphytes and organic and mineral particles, then rinsed in distilled water, and then stored at −20°C until analysis.

Information about Hg concentration in benthic macrofauna was presented by Jędruch et al. [29, 30] and Bełdowska et al. [31]. Samples were collected between 2011 and 2013 using a manual Van Veen grab sampler. In order to separate the benthic organisms, samples of marine sediments were sieved through a 0.5 mm mesh. Live biological material was placed in containers with sea water in situ and transported to the laboratory where they were stored at −20°C until analysis.

The Hg concentration in herring, sprat, and cod from the southern Baltic Sea was obtained from the study by Polak-Juszczak [32]. Samples were collected from 1994 to 2003. Fish were stored at −20°C until analysis.

Information about Hg concentration in gray seals (*Halichoerus grypus*) was presented by Bełdowska and Falkowska [33]. The studies were conducted in the Polish coastal zone of the Baltic Sea during the years 2001–2011. Seal's tissues were obtained from dead individuals found along the coast.

2.2. Chemical analysis

The Hg concentrations in solid samples were determined via pyrolysis with the atomic absorption technique using a direct mercury analyzer [34]. This technique did not require any sample preparation (e.g. extraction/digestion) which would pose a risk of contamination. The analysis of certified reference materials produced both satisfactory recovery and precision.

Water samples for mercury analysis were oxidized by the addition of BrCl and pre-reduced with hydroxylamine hydrochloride solution 1 h prior to analysis by the cold vapor atomic fluorescence technique, according to USEPA method 1631 [35]. Quality control procedures for water samples included blanks, and water spiked with mercury nitrate produced adequate rates of precision and recovery [11].

2.3. Calculations

The Hg concentration in precipitation was used to calculate wet deposition fluxes:

$$F_{wet} = C \times R \tag{1}$$

where F_{wet} is the wet deposition flux (ng m^{-2}); C is the Hg concentration in precipitation (ng dm^{-3}); and R is the amount of precipitation (mm = dm^3 m^{-2}). The Hg load introduced to the Gulf of Gdańsk with wet deposition was calculated by multiplying the wet deposition flux by the area of the Gulf of Gdańsk (4940 km^2).

The Hg dry deposition fluxes were calculated using the formula previously described by Seinfeld and Pandis [36]:

$$F_{dry} = C \times V_d \tag{2}$$

where F_{dry} is the dry deposition flux of Hg (pg m^{-2} s^{-1}); C is the Hg concentration in aerosols (pg m^{-3}); and V_d is the deposition velocity (m s^{-1}). Deposition velocity was not measured during sampling. Therefore, this value was taken from the literature [37, 38] and was 0.005 m s^{-1}. The Hg load introduced to the Gulf of Gdańsk with dry deposition was calculated by multiplying the dry deposition flux by the area of the Gulf of Gdańsk and time of sampling.

The Hg concentration in river water at cross sections close to the river mouth was used to calculate annual Hg load transported into the sea:

$$L_r = C\,Q \tag{3}$$

where L_r is the Hg load (kg s^{-1}); C is the Hg concentration in the river water (μg m^{-3}); and Q is the water flow during sampling (m^3 s^{-1}). The annual Hg load was calculated assuming linear variability in time periods between measurements [39].

The Hg load associated with coastal erosion was calculated based on information presented by Bełdowska et al. [12]. The Hg load form the 1 km long section of the cliff (kg $year^{-1}$) was multiplied by the total length of the cliff sections in the area of the Gulf of Gdańsk (36 km).

The Hg load transported to the sea by the seeping groundwater was estimated by multiplying the Hg concentration in groundwater measured in the Puck Bay [18] by the submarine groundwater discharge rate to the Gulf of Gdańsk (0.07 km^3) [40].

Taking into account the annual air-water flux estimated by Wängberg et al. [41] and data presented by Marks and Bełdowska [42], the Hg load re-emitted from the Gulf of Gdańsk to the atmosphere was calculated.

The yearly Hg sedimentation flux presented by Bełdowski et al. [23] was used to calculate the load of mercury deposited in the Gulf of Gdańsk sediments.

Based on the model calculations [43], the export flux of water from the gulf was estimated. This value was assumed to be equivalent to the volume of water introduced into the gulf by rivers. The outflow of Hg from the Gulf of Gdańsk was calculated by multiplying this volume of water by the Hg concentration measured in the profile at the Gdańsk Deep [20, 21].

The Hg load in the Gulf of Gdańsk water was calculated by multiplying the median values of the Hg concentration in the open water of the gulf [20, 21] and the volume of water in the gulf [4, 5].

Based on the mean Hg concentration in the two types of sediment (sandy and silty), their wetness [24], density [44], and surface of the bottom of each type, the load of Hg deposited in the upper layer of the sediments (0–5 cm) in the Gulf of Gdańsk was estimated.

The amount of Hg bound to the phytoplankton was estimated by multiplying the median of the Hg concentration in phytoplankton in the coastal zone of the Gulf of Gdańsk [25] by the mean phytoplankton biomass in the Gulf [26, 45] and the volume of the water to a depth of 20 meters (where phytoplankton occurs most abundantly).

Taking into account the median of the Hg concentration in zooplankton in the coastal zone of the Gulf of Gdańsk [27], the mean zooplankton biomass in the Gulf [45] and the volume of water in the Gulf [4, 5], the Hg pool in zooplankton was estimated.

The calculation of the Hg load accumulated in macrophytobenthic plants was carried out based on the research conducted by Bełdowska et al. [28] (the Hg concentration in macrophytobenthos), Saniewski and Zalewska [46] (biomass of particular macrophytobenthic plants from the Gulf of Gdańsk) and the area on which these plants occur [4].

The amount of Hg accumulated in macrozoobenthos in the Gulf of Gdańsk was estimated based on the research conducted by Jędruch et al. [29, 30] (the Hg concentration in macrozoobenthos) and Włodarska-Kowalczuk et al. [47] (biomass of particular macrozoobenthic organisms from the Gulf of Gdańsk) and the area on which these organisms occur [4]. Jędruch et al. [29, 30] observed that the macrozoobenthos occurred most abundantly up to a depth of 80 m as well as the Hg concentration in macrozoobenthic organisms was dependent on the type of bottom. Therefore, the bottom area of the Gulf of Gdańsk to a depth of 80 m (3350 km^2) was divided into two types: bottom covered by macrophytobenthos (100 km^2) and bottom not covered by macrophytobenthos (3250 km^2) [Jędruch, personal comm.].

The fish resources of the Gulf of Gdańsk have not yet been reliably estimated. However, information about the biomass of the most common caught fish was available. Therefore, the Hg load exported from the sea with the fish was calculated by multiplying the median values of the Hg concentration in the particular species of the most commonly caught fish [32, 33] and the biomass of these fish [48].

Taking into account the median Hg concentration in the muscle [33], the wetness of the tissue (55%), the average weight of the gray seal (250 kg), and the size of population in the Gulf of Gdańsk [49], the load of Hg accumulated in the gray seals was estimated.

3. External sources and sinks of mercury in the Gulf of Gdańsk

An important source of mercury in the sea is atmospheric deposition. The Hg load introduced into the Gulf of Gdańsk with wet and dry deposition was 17.7 kg $year^{-1}$ and 9.5 kg $year^{-1}$, respectively (**Figure 2**) [10–12, 16]. The inflow of Hg with precipitation dominated in the warm season (May–September), while during the heating season (October-April) dry deposition of mercury associated with aerosols was predominant [10, 11, 16]. The key role in Hg dry deposition was played by the concentration of mercury bound in aerosols, while the particle deposition velocity was of marginal significance [10, 16]. Hg wet deposition flux depended mainly on the amount of precipitation. There was a significant statistical relationship between Hg wet deposition flux and the Hg concentration in the precipitation, only in the warm season [11, 16].

Another important source of Hg in the sea is riverine input. The average annual Hg load carried out into the Gulf of Gdańsk by rivers was estimated to be 200 kg (**Figure 2**) [12–16]. The riverine input of Hg to the Gulf varied between 180 and 220 kg per year [12–16]. A total of 99% of Hg carried out by the rivers was transported by the Vistula (average water flow 1047 $m^3 s^{-1}$), the longest river that flows into the Baltic Sea [6]. The small rivers (average water flow $< 5 m^3 s^{-1}$) provided about 2 kg of Hg [13, 15, 16]. The Hg load transported by rivers to the

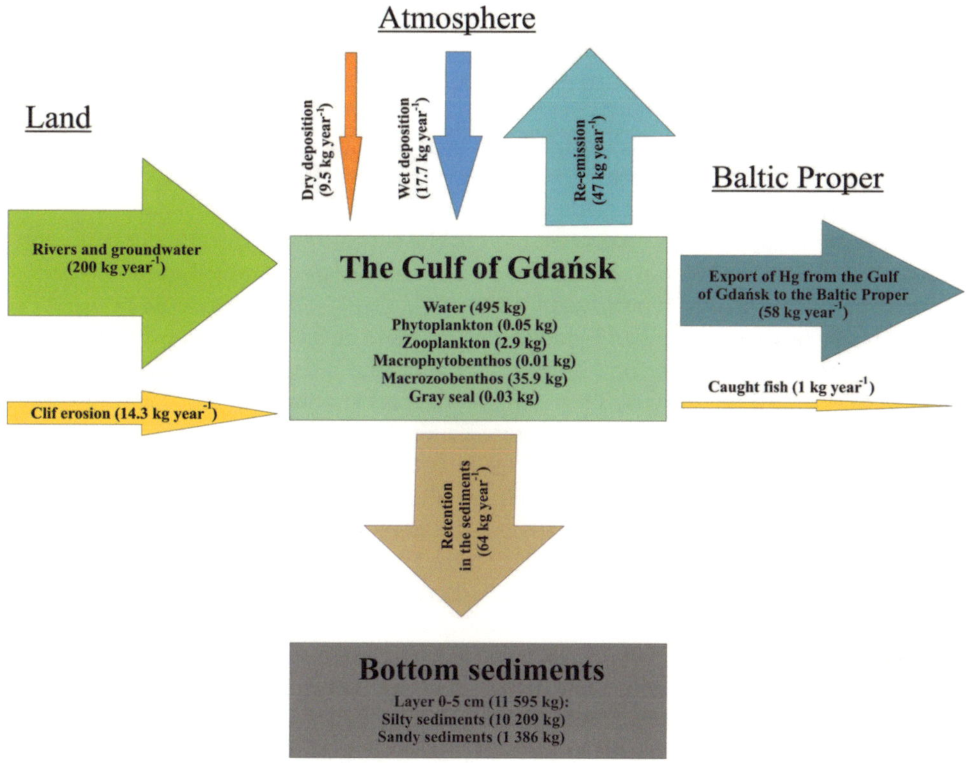

Figure 2.
The mass balance of mercury in the Gulf of Gdańsk.

sea depended on the amount of precipitation and retention capacity of the catchment. In areas of natural character, only 10–30% atmospheric Hg deposited to the catchment outflow from the soil to the river [13, 16, 50, 51]. However, in areas where the catchment was transformed by humans (fields and urban and industrialized areas), Hg outflow was considerably greater than in the natural areas and may have reached up to 65% [13, 16, 52–54]. Saniewska and colleagues [13] showed that in urbanized and agricultural areas, river water was two to three times more polluted with mercury than in the forests. This was influenced not only by the increased Hg outflow from the catchment, but also by the inflow of Hg from anthropogenic sources (e.g. combustion of fossil fuels and point sources). In this area, Hg is emitted into the atmosphere. Consequently, more Hg could be deposited in the catchment and then could be washed out to river water [13, 16, 17]. The Hg load transported by rivers to the sea depended on the river flow [13–16]. This was particularly visible during floods, downpours, and thaws, when river flow was much higher than the average value. At that time, water pours out of the riverbed, which causes local flooding and increased soil erosion [13–16]. During high flow, the Hg daily outflow from the catchment could increase over tenfold than during the period with average [13–16]. This was clearly visible during the Vistula flood of 2010. During the month of the flood, over 1197 kg of mercury flew into the Gulf of Gdańsk, which accounted for 75% of the Hg load transported through 2010 with the Vistula water [14]. During the flood, a very large load of dissolved mercury (around 314 kg) reached the sea. This can have a negative impact on the marine environment, especially on organisms inhabiting river estuaries [14].

An important source of mercury in the Gulf of Gdańsk, usually neglected during the creation of the mass balance of Hg in aquatic ecosystems, is the coastal erosion. Bełdowska et al. [12] estimated that the 1-km long section of the cliff was responsible for the introduction of 0.4 kg of mercury into the sea every year. The total length of the cliff sections in the area of the Gulf of Gdańsk is 36 km. This allows estimating that due to the coastal erosion about 14.3 kg Hg $year^{-1}$ was transported to the sea (**Figure 2**) [12]. A large Hg load introduced through the cliff abrasion into the sea as well as the labile form of mercury, which predominated in the material [19], makes it necessary to understand the consequences of the process for the marine food chain.

In recent years, attention has been paid to the submarine groundwater discharge as a source of mercury in the seas and oceans. The average dissolved mercury concentration in the seeping groundwater was 0.6 ng dm^{-3} [17]. Submarine groundwater discharge rate to the Gulf of Gdańsk was assessed at 0.07 km^3 [40]. The Hg load to the Gulf was estimated to be 42 g $year^{-1}$. This value is negligible in the Hg mass balance in the Gulf of Gdańsk. This is due to the fact that in this case, groundwater was characterized by lower concentrations of Hg than the sea water [17].

Mercury in the sea may also come from point sources such as municipal wastewater treatment plants, industrial plants or fish farms, etc. In the case of the Gulf of Gdańsk, point sources located in the coastal zone were of little importance in the transport of mercury to the sea [55]. This was also confirmed by HELCOM [6]. However, it should be emphasized that contaminants transported this way may adversely affect adjacent ecosystems.

Some part of Hg present in the sea can be re-emitted into the atmosphere. Wängberg et al. [41] estimated that in the southern Baltic, an annual re-emission flux of Hg was equal 9.5 μg m^{-2} $year^{-1}$. It was calculated that approximately 47 kg Hg may be re-emitted from the Gulf of Gdańsk every year (**Figure 2**). This value was 1.7 as high as Hg atmospheric deposition; however, it could still be underestimated. The value of the re-emission flux depends on the weather conditions [41, 42, 56, 57]. The research was conducted in calm conditions, while stormy weather increased emission of both gases and aerosols from the water to the atmosphere. Therefore, detailed studies are necessary to allow an accurate estimation of the re-emission flux of Hg.

Sediments are important sink of Hg in the sea. According to Bełdowski et al. [23], the net mercury input, calculated on the basis of sedimentation rate and concentration in the uppermost sediments, was estimated at 1.3 ng cm^{-2} $year^{-1}$. It follows that every year, about 64 kg of mercury was retained in the sediments (**Figure 2**).

On the basis of the water balance in the Gulf of Gdańsk, the export flux of Hg from the Gulf to the Baltic Proper was estimated. Based on the model [43], it was calculated that the annual export of water from the Gulf of Gdańsk was about 32 km^3. This value was obtained from the difference between the outflow of water from the Gulf to the Baltic Proper and inflow of water from the Baltic Proper to the Gulf. Considering the Hg concentration measured in the profile at the Gdańsk Deep [20, 21], it was estimated that the export of Hg from the Gulf of Gdańsk to the Baltic Proper was about 58 kg $year^{-1}$ (**Figure 2**). It follows that the Gulf was a source of Hg to the sea.

Herring (*Clupea harengus*), sprat (*Sprattus sprattus*), cod (*Gadus morhua*), and flounder (*Platichthys flesus*) are the most frequently caught fish in the Polish part of the Baltic Sea (**Table 1**) [48]. Of the fish caught, the lowest Hg concentration was measured in the sprat, and the highest in flounder (**Table 1**) [32, 33]. The Hg load associated with the caught fish was dependent on the biomass of fish. Approximately 52,796 tons of fish were caught annually in the Gulf of Gdańsk [48]. The highest Hg load was accumulated in the sprat (which accounts to 78% of the total fish biomass taken out), which constituted 61% of the Hg being carried out of the sea with fish (**Table 1**). On the basis of these data, the load of Hg exported from the sea within caught fish was estimated at 937 g (**Figure 2**).

Group	Median of Hg concentration [32, 33] (μg g^{-1})	Mass of caught fish [48] (Mg)	Hg load (g)
Sprat (*Sprattus sprattus*)	0.014	40,442	566.2
Herring (*Clupea harengus*)	0.025	5279	132.0
Cod (*Gadus morhua*)	0.034	4329	147.2
Flounder (*Platichthys flesus*)	0.054	1689	91.2

Table 1.
The Hg load accumulated in the caught fish from the Gulf of Gdańsk.

4. Mercury in different environmental compartments in the Gulf of Gdańsk

The surface water of the offshore part of the Gulf of Gdańsk was characterized by low Hg concentrations (< 2 ng dm^{-3}), which was typical for the Baltic Proper [13–15, 20–23, 58, 59]. The major factor influencing mercury distribution in the water column was suspended matter. Therefore, the Hg concentration was higher in the areas of the density stratification (thermo- and halocline) and in the layer of maximum chlorophyll *a* concentration than in surface water [20, 21]. Higher concentration of Hg in the water in comparison with the offshore water was measured in the vicinity of the coastline—near the industrialized shore as well as in the area of the river mouths; however, the median of the Hg concentration in those areas was still relatively low (< 8 ng dm^{-3}) compared to coastal zones in different parts of the world [60, 61]. Based on the median values of the Hg concentration in the open water of the Gulf of Gdańsk (1.7 ng dm^{-3}) and the volume of water in the Gulf (291.2 km^3) the total amount of Hg in this water body was estimated at 495 kg (**Figure 2**).

In the Gulf of Gdańsk, 4–79% (average 27%) of Hg in sea water was bound to suspended matter [15, 20–22]. This is a relatively high value compared to ocean water, where suspended mercury usually constitutes less than 20% [61, 62]. This is due to the specific properties of the Baltic Sea—low salinity and high content of organic matter (both DOC and POC) in the sea water [63, 64]. Therefore, in this region, suspended particulate matter (SPM) plays a particularly important role in Hg cycling—it acts as the carrier for mercury in the marine environment [20–22]. Organic matter transports Hg toward greater depths and accelerates its sedimentation to the benthic sediments. Taking into account the total amount of Hg in the Gulf of Gdańsk (495 kg) and percentage of Hg bound to suspended matter (27%), it was estimated that about 134 kg Hg in the Gulf was presented in the particulate form.

According to Jędruch et al. [24], the Hg concentration in the sediments varied in a wide range (1.0–325.3 ng g^{-1}). However, this large difference resulted from the properties of the sediments—silty sediments were characterized by much higher Hg concentration (98.8 ng g^{-1}) than sandy one (7.3 ng g^{-1}) [24]. Based on the mean Hg concentration in the two types of sediments, the surface of the bottom and density of each (**Table 2**), it was estimated that the load of Hg deposited in the upper layer of the sediments (0–5 cm) in the Gulf of Gdańsk was 11,595 kg (**Figure 2**). It is worth mentioning that 88% of this load was deposited in silty sediments. Therefore, bottom sediments should be considered as the important Hg reservoir in the sea.

Due to the fact that mercury accumulates and biomagnifies in the marine trophic chain, aquatic organisms should also be considered as Hg reservoir. The median of the Hg concentration in phytoplankton in the coastal zone of the Gulf of Gdańsk was 51 ng g^{-1} [25]. The values depended both on the quantity and species

Type of the sediments	Hg concentration [24] (ng g^{-1})	Surface [4] (km^2)	Density [44] (g cm^{-3})	Wetness [24](%)	Hg load (kg)
Silty sediment	98.8 (38.0–325.3)	3124	2.45	73	10,209
Sandy sediment	7.3 (1.0–29.0)	1816	2.55	18	1386

Table 2.
The Hg load deposited in the upper layer of the sediments (0–5 cm) in the Gulf of Gdańsk.

composition of phytoplankton and on mercury sources in the Gulf [25, 26]. The mean phytoplankton biomass in the Gulf of Gdańsk was assumed to be 85 mg m^{-3} [26, 45] and the volume of the water to a depth of 20 m (where phytoplankton occurs most abundantly) was 10.9 km^3 [4]. This information allowed to estimate the amount of Hg bound to the phytoplankton at 47 g (**Figure 2**).

Slightly higher Hg concentrations than in phytoplankton were measured in zooplankton (66 ng g^{-1}) [27]. The Hg concentration in zooplankton presented by Bełdowska and Mudrak-Cegiołka [27] was about 4-fold lower than that measured 20 years earlier by Boszke et al. [65]. This was the result of a systematic reduction of the Hg emission into the environment [6, 66], which in turn caused a decrease of metal concentrations in the water as well as in marine organisms. Taking into account the mean zooplankton biomass in the Gulf of Gdańsk (150 mg m^{-3}; [45]) and the volume of water in the Gulf (291.2 km^3), the Hg pool in zooplankton was estimated at 2.9 kg (**Figure 2**).

Lower Hg concentrations than in plankton were measured in macrophytobenthic plants [28, 29]. The Hg concentration in macrophytobenthos depended on the species and the area of research. The highest Hg concentration was measured in the red algae, while the lowest in the brown algae (**Table 3**). Similar to zooplankton, also in case of phytobenthic plant, the Hg concentrations were found to be much lower than those determined in 1995–1998 in the Puck Bay region [65]. Based on the research conducted by Bełdowska et al. [28] (the Hg concentration in macrophytobenthos) and Saniewski and Zalewska [46] (biomass of particular organism), the Hg load accumulated in macrophytobenthic plants was estimated at 13.9 g (**Table 3**). This value was very low compared to the Hg load presented in zooplankton organisms and was unnoticeable in the Hg mass balance in the Gulf (**Figure 2**). The highest Hg load among macrophytes was accumulated in the vascular plants (8.2 g) (**Table 3**). This group also had one of the highest biomass among discussed organisms. Therefore, subsequent rise in biomass of vascular plants, which has been observed in the Gulf of Gdańsk in recent years, may play a significant role in increasing concentration of this metal in more advanced organisms.

The Hg concentration measured in macrozoobenthos in the Gulf of Gdańsk varied in a wide range (**Table 4**) [29–31]. The Hg level in macrozoobenthos was dependent on its trophic preferences as well as biotic (i.e. primary production and

Group	Hg concentration [28] (ng g^{-1})	Biomass [46] (g m^2)	Surface [4] (km^2)	Hg load (g)
Green algae (*Chlorophyta*)	10.1 (0.8–37.1)	0.668	20.4	0.1
Brown algae (*Phaeophyta*)	5.2 (4.3–6.8)	41.860	20.4	4.4
Red algae (*Rhodophyta*)	11.0 (1.3–43.3)	5.391	20.4	1.2
Vascular plant (*Spermatophyta*)	8.3 (1.3–57.2)	12.497	78.6	8.2

Table 3.
The Hg load accumulated in the macrophytobenthic plants in the Gulf of Gdańsk.

	Group	Hg concentration [29, 30] (ng g^{-1})	Biomass [47] (g m^2)	Surface [4] (km^2)	Hg load (kg)
Bottom not covered by macrophytobenthos	Bivalvia	46.0 (7.4–123.3)	14.6	3250	2.2
	Crustacea	128.1 (8.2–410.2)	61.1	3250	25.4
	Gastropoda	9.8 (26.2–110.5)	14.7	3250	0.5
	Polychaeta	34.0 (9.3–157.4)	48.3	3250	5.3
	Oligochaeta	36.3 (8.7–223.4)	9.6	3250	1.1
	Insect larvae	50.3 (10.9–97.9)	1.8	3250	0.3
	sum				**34.8**
Bottom covered by macrophytobenthos	Bivalvia	44.1 (12.7–76.9)	22.2	100	0.1
	Crustacea	49.0 (8.5–213.7)	79.2	100	0.4
	Gastropoda	58.0 (30.7–185.6)	69.0	100	0.4
	Polychaeta	21.6 (12.6–39.7)	99.6	100	0.2
	Oligochaeta	21.8 (8.6–521.2)	13.2	100	0.0
	Nemertea	59.2 (23.2–460.2)	3.0	100	0.0
	Insect larvae	17.9 (14.9–177.9)	13.8	100	0.0
	sum				**1.1**

Table 4.
The Hg load accumulated in the macrozoobenthos in the Gulf of Gdańsk.

biomass of fauna) and abiotic (salinity, ion composition and Eh) factors. The Hg concentration in macrozoobenthos measured in the Gulf of Gdańsk was in the same range like those determined by Boszke et al. in 1995–1998 in the Puck Bay [65]. This indicates that sediments—habitat of macrozoobenthos—need much more time to reduce the Hg than sea water [67]. The amount of Hg accumulated in macrozoobenthos in the Gulf of Gdańsk based on the research conducted by Jędruch et al. [29, 30] (the Hg concentration in macrozoobenthos), Włodarska-Kowalczuk et al. [47] (biomass of particular macrozoobenthic organisms from the Gulf of Gdańsk), and the area on which these organisms occur [4] was estimated at 35.9 kg (**Figure 2**, **Table 4**). A total of 96% of this load was contained in the organisms dwelling at the bottom not covered by macrophytobenthos (**Table 4**). The organisms that were most responsible for accumulation of Hg were Crustacea, while Gastropoda and insect larvae were of a marginal importance (**Table 4**).

The fish resources of the Gulf of Gdańsk have not yet been reliably estimated. Therefore, estimation of the Hg load associated with the fish was impossible.

The gray seal (*Halichoerus grypus*) is a species representing the highest level of the trophic chain, which most frequently occurs in the Gulf of Gdańsk. The size of its population in the Gulf is estimated at 150 specimens [60]. The median Hg concentration in seal's muscle was 1.81 µg g^{-1} [59]. This value was 130-times higher than in sprat, the main diet of seals (**Table 1**). Taking into account the median Hg concentration in the muscle, the wetness of the tissue (55%), the average weight of the gray seal (250 kg), and the size of population in the Gulf of Gdańsk [60], the load of Hg accumulated in the gray seals was estimated at 31 g.

5. Mass balance of mercury in the Gulf of Gdańsk

Every year around 242 kg of mercury was introduced into the Gulf of Gdańsk (**Figure 2**). The most efficient way of Hg transport to the Gulf of Gdańsk was river runoff, which constituted 83% of Hg flowing into the Gulf (**Figure 3**). This is a typical situation for water bodies, where there is a relatively high ratio of catchment area to the surface of the reservoir itself [68]. A similar tendency was observed in the whole Baltic Sea, where 86% of Hg came from surface runoff, while 14% of Hg came from atmospheric deposition [69, 70].

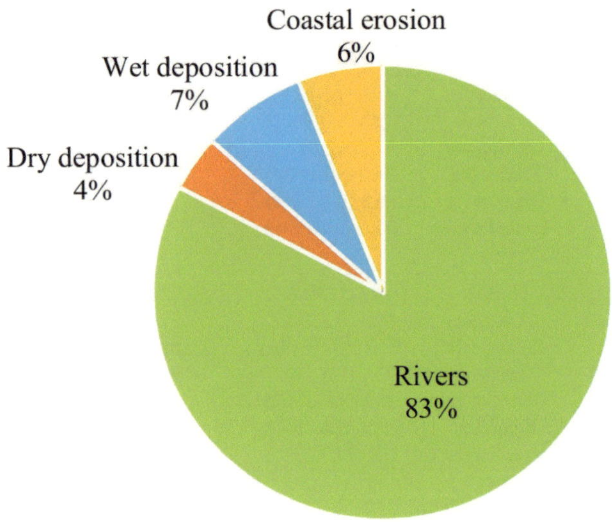

Figure 3.
The percentage share of the main mercury sources in the Gulf of Gdańsk.

The second most important source of Hg in the Gulf of Gdańsk was atmospheric deposition (**Figure 3**). Wet and dry deposition accounts for 7% and 4% of the Hg load reaching the Gulf, respectively. This is a typical situation, because wet deposition of mercury prevails in moderate latitudes. Dry deposition usually accounts for less than 30% of the Hg atmospheric input. Atmospheric deposition introduced much lower Hg load than the rivers; however, considering that the "atmospheric" Hg is much more bioavailable than "riverine" Hg, it played a crucial role in incorporating Hg into the marine trophic chain.

Another source of mercury in the Gulf of Gdańsk, which should be taken into account during the creation of mass balance of Hg is the coastal erosion. In the Gulf of Gdańsk, it accounts for only 6% of the Hg load reaching the sea (**Figure 3**). However, in regions where there are no such large rivers as the Vistula, the significance of this source will increase considerably [12, 19].

Point sources and submarine groundwater discharge have a negligible impact on the Hg load of this metal getting to the Gulf of Gdańsk.

Hg transported to the Gulf only in a small extent reached the open sea water (58 kg—24%). Consequently, the Gulf of Gdańsk should be treated as a cleansing zone for the Baltic Proper. Most Hg was removed from the water through the sedimentation of the metal bound to suspended particulate matter and its deposition into the sediments. This process caused that the bottom sediments are the main Hg reservoir in the Gulf of Gdańsk (**Figure 2**). The third most important process decreasing the Hg load in the Gulf of Gdańsk was re-emission of this metal to the atmosphere (**Figure 2**) [41, 42]. This indicated that seawater was an important source of mercury to the coastal atmosphere. Fishing as a process of removing mercury from the sea can be omitted in the mercury mass balance in the Gulf of Gdańsk (**Figure 2**).

6. Conclusions

The main sources of mercury in the Gulf of Gdańsk were river runoff, atmospheric deposition, and coastal erosion, while the most important processes that reduced Hg load in the Gulf were deposition of Hg to the sediments, re-emission of Hg to the atmosphere, and export to the Baltic Proper. The resultant of all discussed processes was the mercury load accumulated in water and marine organisms. It was estimated that 495 kg of Hg was contained in the sea water. About 12 times smaller load was incorporated into marine organisms. The Hg concentrations in the different environmental compartments in the aquatic ecosystem of the Gulf of Gdańsk measured in 2010s were lower than measured 20 years earlier [65]. This was the result of a reduction of the Hg emission into the environment [6, 66]. This makes that nowadays the Hg concentration in the Gulf of Gdańsk are similar to values observed in different unpolluted coastal regions [60, 61]. However, climate change occurring in the southern Baltic region could change this tendency [71, 72]. On the one hand, the forecasts of climate change in this region anticipate an increase in total annual precipitation as well as an increase in the intensity and frequency of extreme phenomena i.e. storms and floods [31, 73]. These processes lead to the washing out of Hg from both the atmosphere (wet deposition) and from land (river runoff and coastal erosion) [12, 13–16, 19, 22]. In consequence, in the next few decades we can expect an uncontrolled increase in the Hg load transported into the sea. On the other hand, climate warming (especially mild winters without the ice cover) stimulates the growth of marine organisms during the prolonged vegetative season (more frequent blooms and higher biomass). Consequently, this process increases the Hg accumulation by organisms and an increase of the Hg load introduced into the marine trophic chain. Research conducted by Bełdowska et al. [26, 31] indicated that the mean annual Hg pool in phytoplankton, macrophytobenthos, and macrozoobenthos communities in a year without icing was higher compared to an estimated previous year in which the icing period lasted approximately 90 days (by 30%, 30% and 25%, respectively). This can have a negative impact on the marine environment, especially on organisms inhabiting river estuaries.

Acknowledgements

This work was supported by the National Science Centre (grant number 2014/13/B/ST10/02807).

Conflict of interest

The author declares that she has no conflict of interest.

Author details

Dominika Saniewska
Faculty of Oceanography and Geography, Institute of Oceanography, University of Gdańsk, Gdynia, Poland

*Address all correspondence to: dominika.saniewska@gmail.com

References

[1] Scheuhammer AM, Meyer MW, Sandheinrich MB, Murray MW. Effects of environmental methylmercury on the health of wild birds, mammals, and fish. Ambio. 2007;**36**(1):12-18. DOI: 10.1579/0044-7447(2007)36[12,EOEMOT]2.0.CO;2

[2] Boening DW. Ecological effects, transport, and fate of mercury: A general review. Chemosphere. 2000;**40**:1335-1351. DOI: 10.1016/S0045-6535(99)00283-0

[3] Falandysz J, Chwir A, Wyrzykowska B. Total mercury contamination of some fish species in the firth of Vistula and the lower Vistula River, Poland. Polish Journal of Environmental Studies. 2000;**9**:335-339

[4] Majewski A. Gulf of Gdańsk. Warszawa: Geological Publ; 1990. 500 pp. (in Polish)

[5] Łukawska-Matuszewska K, Bolałek J. Spatial distribution of phosphorus forms in sediments in the Gulf of Gdańsk (southern Baltic Sea). Continental Shelf Research. 2008;**28**(7):977-990. DOI: 10.1016/j.csr.2008.01.009

[6] HELCOM. Towards a tool for quantifying anthropogenic pressures and potential impacts on the Baltic Sea marine environment: A background document on the method, data and testing of the Baltic Sea pressure and impact indices. In: Baltic Sea Environment Proceedings. Helsinki, Finland: Helsinki Commission; 2010. p. 125

[7] Brzezińska A. The occurrence of mercury in the southern Baltic Sea. Oceanologia. 1984;**18**:109-116

[8] Wrembel HZ. Mercury in the Baltic Sea. Słupsku: Akademia Pedagogiczna; 1997. pp. 6-177. (in Polish)

[9] Zaborska A, Siedlewicz G, Szymczycha B, Dzierzbicka-Glowacka L, Pazdro K. Legacy and emerging pollutants in the Gulf of Gdańsk (southern Baltic Sea)—Loads and distribution revisited. Marine Pollution Bulletin. 2019;**139**:238-255. DOI: 10.1016/j.marpolbul.2018.11.060

[10] Bełdowska M, Saniewska D, Falkowska L, Lewandowska A. Mercury in particulate matter over the polish zone of the southern Baltic Sea. Atmospheric Environment. 2012;**46**:397-404. DOI: 10.1016/j.atmosenv.2011.09.046

[11] Saniewska D, Bełdowska M, Bełdowski J, Falkowska L. Mercury in precipitation at an urbanised coastal zone of the Baltic Sea (Poland). Ambio. 2014;**43**(7):871-877. DOI: 10.1007/s13280-014-0494-y

[12] Bełdowska M, Jędruch A, Łęczyński L, Saniewska D, Kwasigroch U. Coastal erosion as a source of mercury into the marine environment along the polish Baltic shore. Environmental Science and Pollution Research. 2016;**23**(16):16372-16382. DOI: 10.1007/s11356-016-6753-7

[13] Saniewska D, Bełdowska M, Bełdowski J, Saniewski M, Szubska M, Romanowski A, et al. The impact of land use and season on the riverine transport of mercury into the marine coastal zone. Environmental Monitoring and Assessment. 2014;**186**(11):7593-7604. DOI: 10.1007/s10661-014-3950-z

[14] Saniewska D, Bełdowska M, Bełdowski J, Jędruch A, Saniewski M, Falkowska L. Mercury loads into the sea associated with extreme flooding. Environmental Pollution. 2014;**191**:93-100. DOI: 10.1016/j.envpol.2014.04.003

[15] Saniewska D, Bełdowska M, Bełdowski J, Saniewski M, Gębka K, Szubska M, et al. Impact of intense rains

and flooding on mercury riverine input to the coastal zone. Marine Pollution Bulletin. 2018;**127**:593-602. DOI: 10.1016/j.marpolbul.2017.12.058

[16] Bełdowska M, Saniewska D, Falkowska L. Factors influencing variability of mercury input to the southern Baltic Sea. Marine Pollution Bulletin. 2014;**86**:283-290. DOI: 10.1016/j.marpolbul.2014.07.004

[17] Gębka K, Bełdowska M, Saniewska D, Kuliński K, Bełdowski J. Watershed characteristics and climate factors effect on the temporal variability of mercury in the southern Baltic Sea rivers. Journal of Environmental Sciences. 2018;**68**:55-64. DOI: 10.1016/j.jes.2017.11.030

[18] Szymczycha B, Miotk M, Pempkowiak J. Submarine groundwater discharge as a source of mercury in the bay of Puck, the southern Baltic Sea. Water, Air, and Soil Pollution. 2013;**224**:1542-1557. DOI: 10.1007/s11270-013-1542-0

[19] Kwasigroch U, Bełdowska M, Jędruch A, Saniewska D. Coastal erosion—A "new" land-based source of labile mercury to the marine environment. Environmental Science and Pollution Research. 2018;**25**(28):28682-28694. DOI: 10.1007/s11356-018-2856-7

[20] Saniewska D, Bełdowska M, Bełdowski J, Saniewski M, Kwaśniak J, Falkowska L. Distribution of mercury in different environmental compartments in the aquatic ecosystem of the coastal zone of the southern Baltic Sea. Journal of Environmental Sciences. 2010;**22**(8):1144-1150. DOI: 10.1016/S1001-0742(09)60230-8

[21] Murawiec D, Gajecka A, Bełdowska M, Falkowska L. Investigation on mercury concentration levels in coastal and offshore waters of the Gulf of Gdansk. Oceanological and Hydrobiological Studies. 2007;**36**:83-97

[22] Jędruch A, Kwasigroch U, Bełdowska M, Kuliński K. Mercury in suspended matter of the Gulf of Gdańsk: Origin, distribution and transport at the land–sea interface. Marine Pollution Bulletin. 2017;**118**(1-2):354-367. DOI: 10.1016/j.marpolbul.2017.03.019

[23] Bełdowski J, Miotk M, Pempkowiak J. Mercury fluxes through the sediment water interface and bioavailability of mercury in southern Baltic Sea sediments. Oceanologia. 2009;**51**:263-285. DOI: 10.5697/oc.51-2.263

[24] Jędruch A, Bełdowski J, Bełdowska M. Long-term changes and distribution of mercury concentrations in surface sediments of the Gdansk Basin (southern Baltic Sea). Journal of Soils and Sediments. 2015;**15**(12):2487-2497. DOI: 10.1007/s11368-015-1148-9

[25] Bełdowska M, Kobos J. The variability of Hg concentration and composition of marine phytoplankton. Environmental Science and Pollution Research. 2018;**25**(30):30366-30374. DOI: 10.1007/s11356-018-2948-4

[26] Bełdowska M, Kobos J. Mercury concentration in phytoplankton in response to warming of an autumn–winter season. Environmental Pollution. 2016;**215**:38-47. DOI: 10.1016/j.envpol.2016.05.002

[27] Bełdowska M, Mudrak-Cegiołka S. Mercury concentration variability in the zooplankton of the southern Baltic coastal zone. Progress in Oceanography. 2017;**159**:73-85. DOI: 10.1016/j.pocean.2017.09.009

[28] Bełdowska M, Jędruch A, Słupkowska J, Saniewska D, Saniewski M. Macrophyta as a vector of contemporary and historical mercury from the marine environment to the trophic web. Environmental Science and Pollution Research. 2015;**22**(7):5228-5240. DOI: 10.1007/s11356-014-4003-4

[29] Jędruch A, Bełdowska M, Ziółkowska M. The role of benthic macrofauna in the trophic transfer of mercury in a low-diversity temperate coastal ecosystem (Puck lagoon, southern Baltic Sea). Environmental Monitoring and Assessment. 2019;**191**:137-172. DOI: 10.1007/s10661-019-7257-y

[30] Jędruch A, Bełdowska M, Graca B. Seasonal variation in accumulation of mercury in the benthic macrofauna in a temperate coastal zone (Gulf of Gdańsk). Ecotoxicology and Environmental Safety. 2018;**164**:305-316. DOI: 10.1016/j.ecoenv.2018.08.040

[31] Bełdowska M, Jędruch A, Zgrundo A, Ziółkowska M, Graca B, Gębka K. The influence of cold season warming on the mercury pool in coastal benthic organisms. Estuarine, Coastal and Shelf Science. 2016;**171**:99-105. DOI: 10.1016/j.ecss.2016.01.033

[32] Polak-Juszczak L. Temporal trends in the bioaccumulation of trace metals in herring, sprat, and cod from the southern Baltic Sea in the 1994-2003 period. Chemosphere. 2009;**76**(10):1334-1339. DOI: 10.1016/j.chemosphere.2009.06.030

[33] Bełdowska M, Falkowska L. Mercury in marine fish, mammals, seabirds, and human hair in the coastal zone of the southern Baltic. Water, Air, and Soil Pollution. 2016;**227**:52. DOI: 10.1007/s11270-015-2735-5

[34] Saniewska D, Bełdowska M. Mercury fractionation in soil and sediment samples using thermo-desorption method. Talanta. 2017;**168**:152-161

[35] USEPA (US Environmental Protection Agency). Method 1631, Revision E: Mercury in water by oxidation, purge and trap, and cold vapor atomic fluorescence spectrometry. US Environmental Protection Agency, Office of Water 4303, EPA-821-R-02-019; 2002. pp. 1-46

[36] Seinfeld JH, Pandis SN. Atmospheric Chemistry and Physics-From Air Pollution to Climate Change. New York: John Wiley & Sons; 1998

[37] Lamborg CH, Fitzgerald WF, Vandal GM, Rolfhus KR. Atmospheric mercury in northern Wisconsin: Sources and species. Water, Air, and Soil Pollution. 1995;**80**:198-206

[38] Fang F, Wang Q, Liu R, Ma Z, Hao Q. Atmospheric particulate mercury in Changchun City, China. Atmospheric Environment. 2001;**35**:4265-4272

[39] Niemirycz E. Inflow of chemicals with rivers. In: Uścinowicz J, editor. Geochemistry of the Surface Sediments of the Baltic Sea. Warszawa: Państwowy Instytut Geologiczny-Państwowy Instytut Badawczy; 2011. ISBN: 978-83-7538-813-8, pp. 93-113. (in Polish)

[40] Uścinowicz S. Geochemistry of the Surface Sediments of the Baltic Sea. Warszawa: Państwowy Instytut Geologiczny-Państwowy Instytut Badawczy; 2011. ISBN: 978-83-7538-813-8. (in Polish)

[41] Wängberg I, Schmolke S, Schager P, Munthe J, Ebinhaus R, Iverfeldt A. Estimates of air-sea exchange of mercury in the Baltic Sea. Atmospheric Environment. 2001;**35**:5477-5484. DOI: 10.1016/S1352-2310(01)00246-1

[42] Marks R, Bełdowska M. Air-sea exchange of mercury vapour over the Gulf of Gdańsk and southern Baltic Sea. Journal of Marine Systems. 2001;**27**:315-324. DOI: 10.1016/S0924-7963(00)00076-2

[43] Jędrasik J. A model of matter exchange and flow of energy in the Gulf of Gdańsk ecosystem-overview. Oceanological Studies. 1997;**26**:3-20

[44] Jankowska H, Łęczyński L. Bottom sediments. In: Korzeniewski K, editor. The Puck Bay. Gdańsk: University of Gdańsk; 2003. (in Polish)

[45] Krzymiński W. Evaluation of the environmental condition of the Polish Baltic maritime areas during the 2016 year on the background of decade 2006-2015. GIOŚ; 2017. p. 163 (in Polish)

[46] Saniewski M, Zalewska T. Budget of 90Sr in the Gulf of Gdańsk (southern Baltic Sea). Oceanologia. 2018;**60**:256-263. DOI: 10.1016/j.oceano.2017.11.002

[47] Włodarska-Kowalczuk M, Jankowska E, Kotwicki L, Bałazy P. Evidence of season-dependency in vegetation effects on macrofauna in temperate Seagrass meadows (Baltic Sea). PLoS One. 2014;**9**(7):e100788. DOI: 10.1371/journal.pone.0100788

[48] Szostak S, Rakowski M, Budny T. Maritime Fishing Industry in 2011. Gdynia: National Marine Fisheries Research Institute; 2012. 34 pp. (in Polish)

[49] The gray seal [Internet]. Available from: http://www.fokarium.com/newsyfoki/foka%20szara.html [Accessed: January, 02 2019]

[50] Bishop KH, Lee Y-H. Mercury and its effects on environment and biology. In: Sigel A, Sigel H, editors. Metal Ions in Biological Systems. New York: Marcel Dekker; 1997

[51] Driscoll CT, Holsapple J, Schofield CL, Munson R. The chemistry and transport of mercury in a small wetland in the Adirondack region of New York, USA. Biogeochemistry. 1998;**40**:137-146. DOI: 10.1023/A:1005989229089

[52] Eckley CS, Branfireun B. Mercury mobilization in urban stormwater runoff. Science of the Total Environment. 2008;**403**:164-177. DOI: 10.1016/j.scitotenv.2008.05.021

[53] Mason RP, Lawson NM, Sullivan KA. The concentration, speciation and sources of mercury in Chesapeake Bay precipitation. Atmospheric Environment. 1997;**31**:3541-3550. DOI: 10.1016/S1352-2310(97)00206-9

[54] Saniewska D, Gębka K, Bełdowska M, Siedlewicz G, Bełdowski J. Impact of hydrotechnical works on outflow of mercury from the riparian zone to a river and input to the sea. Marine Pollution Bulletin. 2019;**142**:361-376

[55] Saniewska D. Input pathways of mercury to the coastal zone of the Gulf of Gdansk [thesis]. University of Gdańsk; 2013. (in Polish)

[56] Bełdowska M, Zawalich K, Falkowska L, Siudek P, Magulski R. Total gaseous mercury in the area of southern Baltic and in the coastal zone of the Gulf of Gdańsk during spring and autumn. Environment Protection Engineering. 2008;**34**(4):139-144

[57] Costa M, Liss P. Photoreduction and evolution of mercury from seawater. The Science of the Total Environment. 2000;**261**:125-135

[58] Pempkowiak J, Cossa D, Sikora A, Sanjuan J. Mercury in water and sediments of the southern Baltic Sea. The Science of the Total Environment. 1998;**213**((1)–(3)):185-192. DOI: 10.1016/S0048-9697(98)00091-6

[59] Wurl O, Elsholz O, Ebighaus R. On-line determination of total mercury in the Baltic Sea. Analytica Chimica Acta. 2001;**438**((1)–(2)): 245-249. DOI: 10.1016/S0003-2670(01)00918-7

[60] Baeyens W, Leermakers M. Elemental mercury concentrations and formation rates in the Scheldt estuary and the North Sea. Marine Chemistry. 1998;**60**:257-266. DOI: 10.1016/S0304-4203(97)00102-3

[61] Horvat M, Kotnik J, Logar M, Fajon V, Zvonaric T, Pirrone N. Speciation of mercury in surface and deep-sea waters in Mediterranean Sea. Atmospheric Environment. 2003;**37**:93-108. DOI: 10.1016/S1352-2310(03)00249-8

[62] Laurier FJG, Mason RP, Gill GA, Whalin L. Mercury distributions in the North Pacific Ocean-20 years of observations. Marine Chemistry. 2004;**90**:3-19. DOI: 10.1016/j.marchem.2004.02.025

[63] Szymczycha B, Winogradow A, Kuliński K, Kozierowska K, Pempkowiak J. Diurnal and seasonal DOC and POC variability in the land-locked sea. Oceanologia. 2017;**59**(3):379-388. DOI: 10.1016/j.oceano.2017.03.008

[64] Saniewska D, Gębka K, Łukawska-Matuszewska K, Bełdowska M, Wochna A. The effect of land use in the catchment and meteorological conditions on the riverine transport of dissolved organic carbon into the Puck lagoon (southern Baltic). Environmental Monitoring and Assessment. 2018;**190**(9):536. DOI: 10.1007/s10661-018-6857-22018

[65] Boszke L, Siepak J, Falandysz F. Total mercury contamination of selected organisms in bay of Puck, Baltic Sea, Poland. Polish Journal of Environmental Studies. 2003;**12**(3):275-285

[66] HELCOM. The fourth Baltic Sea pollution load compilation (PLC-4). In: Baltic Sea Environment Proceedings. Helsinki, Finland: Helsinki Commission; 2004. p. 93

[67] Bełdowski J, Pempkowiak J. Horizontal and vertical variabilities of mercury concentration and speciation in sediments of the Gdansk Basin, southern Baltic Sea. Chemosphere. 2003;**52**:645-654. DOI: 10.1016/S0045-6535(03)00246-7

[68] Balcom PH, Fitzgerald WF, Vandal GM, Lamborg CH, Rolfhus KR, Langer CS, et al. Mercury sources and cycling in the Connecticut River and Long Island sound. Marine Chemistry. 2004;**90**:53-74. DOI: 10.1016/j.marchem.2004.02.020

[69] Bartnicki J, Gusev A, Aas W, Fagerli H, Valiyaveetil S. Atmospheric supply of nitrogen, lead, cadmium, mercury and dioxines/furanes to the Baltic Sea in 2006. EMEP Centers Joint Report for HELCOM EMEP/MSC-W Technical Report 3/2008

[70] Knuuttila S. Waterborne inputs of heavy metals to the Baltic Sea. HELCOM Indicator Fact Sheet; 2009

[71] Kundzewicz ZW, Matczak P. Natural risks: Mitigation and adaptation. Ecohydrology and Hydrobiology. 2012;**12**(1):3-8. DOI: 10.2478/v10104-012-0005-3

[72] HELCOM. Climate change in the Baltic Sea area: HELCOM thematic assessment in 2013. Baltic Sea Environment Proceedings; 2013. p. 137

[73] Bełdowska M. Review of mercury circulation changes in the coastal zone of southern Baltic Sea. In: Marghany M, editor. Applied Studies of Coastal and Marine Environments. Rijeka, Croatia: Intechopen; 2016. pp. 109-124. DOI: 10.5772/61991

Chapter 7

Metazoan Endoparasites as Biological Indicators of Baltic Cod Biology

Kurt Buchmann

Abstract

The Baltic cod is a substock of the Atlantic cod *Gadus morhua*, and it is divided into two subpopulations (the western and the eastern stock) living in the semi-enclosed Baltic Sea. This brackish water area is receiving high salinity water from the North Sea through the Danish straits (the Great Belt, Øresund, and Little Belt) and freshwater from precipitation and the drainage areas in surrounding countries whereby marked differences with regard to salinity conditions occur in various parts of the area. The biological and hydrographical conditions determine the parasite fauna found in the Baltic cod, and therefore several of the Baltic parasites are biological indicators. Recommended indicator parasites comprise trematodes (*Cryptocotyle lingua*, *Diplostomum spathaceum*, *Lepidapedon elongatum*, *Hemiurus lühei*, *Brachyphallus crenatus*), nematodes (*Hysterothylacium aduncum*, *Contracaecum osculatum*, *Anisakis simplex*, *Pseudoterranova decipiens*, *Capillaria gracilis*), and acanthocephalans (*Echinorhynchus gadi*, *Corynosoma* spp., *Pomphorhynchus laevis*).

Keywords: Baltic cod, parasites, life cycle, ecological indicators

1. Introduction

The Baltic Sea is a dynamic ecosystem composed of zoological and botanical communities continuously exposed to marked changes of salinity, temperature, and oxygen conditions [1]. It is receiving high salinity water from the North Sea through the Danish straits (Great Belt, Øresund, and Little Belt) whereas freshwater is received from precipitation and drainage areas in surrounding countries including Denmark, Sweden, Finland, Russia, Estonia, Latvia, Lithuania, Poland, and Germany whereby highly varying salinity occur in different parts of the basin. One of the main marine fish stocks in the Baltic Sea is a subpopulation of the Atlantic cod (*Gadus morhua*) termed the Baltic cod. It is composed of a western substock (spawning in the western Baltic) and an eastern substock (with a main spawning zone in the Bornholm Basin), and these two fish groups have a mixing zone around the island of Bornholm [2]. The Atlantic cod, when considering its entire area of distribution, is able to carry a long range of parasites (more than 120 species) belonging to many different systematic groups [3]. Many of the metazoan endoparasites have relatively complicated life cycles some of which include invertebrates, fish, birds, or mammals (**Figure 1**). The distribution in the Baltic of these major animal groups is dependent on biological and hydrographical conditions in various salinity zones, and their distribution will to some extent determine the parasite fauna found in the Baltic cod whereby these can

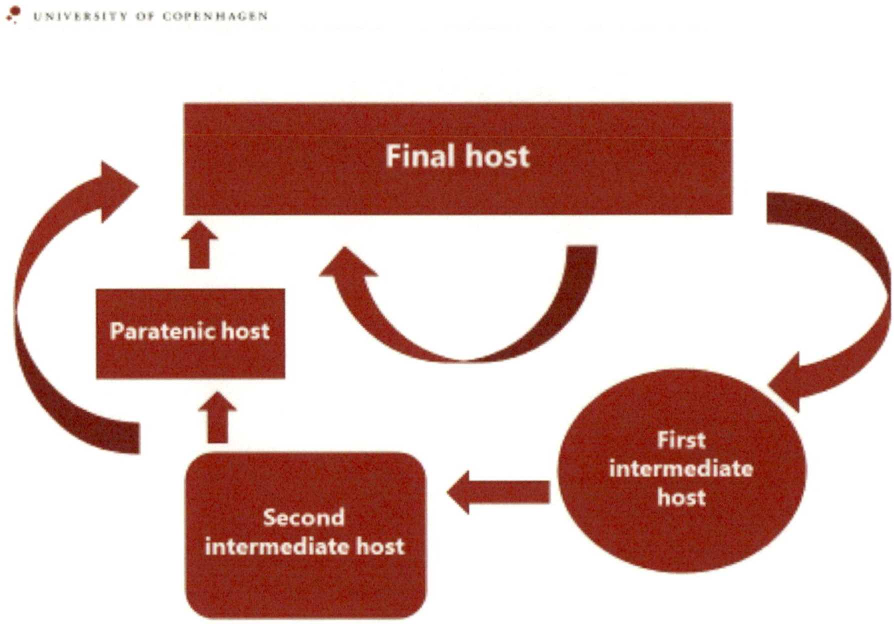

Figure 1.
Diagrammatic presentation of the life cycle of different parasites with inclusion of no, one, or two intermediate hosts and transport hosts (paratenic hosts).

be applied as biological indicators. The use of parasites in fish as indicators has been suggested and documented by numerous authors [4–13]. Although many parasite species display a high degree of host specificity, some parasite species infect a broad variety of fish. The occurrence of fish species other than the cod will therefore add to the overall infection pressure and thereby affect the exposure of Baltic cod to various parasite species with low specificity. Sharing of parasites occurs with important local fish species such as the Baltic salmon (*Salmo salar*), sea trout (*Salmo trutta*), European eel (*Anguilla anguilla*), herring (*Clupea harengus*), sprat (*Sprattus sprattus*), eelpout (*Zoarces viviparus*), flounder (*Platichthys flesus*), plaice (*Pleuronectes platessa*), and turbot (*Scophthalmus maximus*). In addition freshwater species including smelt (*Osmerus eperlanus*), perch (*Perca fluviatilis*), pike (*Esox lucius*), three-spined stickleback (*Gasterosteus aculeatus*), ruffe (*Acerina cernua*), roach (*Rutilus rutilus*), and pikeperch (*Stizostedion lucioperca*) occur with increasing frequency towards the northern parts of the Baltic characterized by low salinity [14]. The invertebrate fauna in the Baltic is highly variable and shifts from a dominance of marine animal species in the western Baltic to freshwater species in the eastern and northern parts of the sea. Of special importance is the presence of potential intermediate hosts such as the marine snail, the common periwinkle *Littorina littorea* which is frequently found in the western Baltic but absent in the eastern Baltic. In contrast, the freshwater snail, *Lymnaea (Radix) peregra*, is absent in the most saline parts of the western Baltic but extremely common in the eastern Baltic [15]. Important invertebrates, besides molluscs, when discussing parasites of fish, are also the copepods, amphipods, and polychaetes because they act as intermediate hosts in several life cycles of parasites found in Baltic fishes. Marine mammals occur in the Baltic, and especially the grey seal (*Halichoerus grypus*) population increase has recently been associated with marked changes in the parasite fauna of cod in the Baltic [13, 16–21]. However, other pinniped species such as ringed seal and harbour seal contribute to some extent in various parts of this brackish water system. A series of fish-eating birds, especially sea gulls, occurring in the Baltic play an important role as final hosts for digeneans and nematodes [14, 15, 22] (**Table 1**).

Parasite	Final host	First intermediate or transport host	Second intermediate or transport host	Paratenic/ transport host	Distribution
Trematodes					
Cryptocotyle lingua	Fish-eating birds	*Littorina littorea*	Fish including cod	NA	Atlantic, western Baltic
Diplostomum spp.	Fish-eating birds	*Radix balthica*	Fish including cod	NA	Freshwaters and eastern Baltic
Brachyphallus crenatus	Fish	*Retusa obtusa*	Copepods	Pelagic fish including clupeids	Atlantic, western Baltic, Central Baltic
Hemiurus luehei	Fish	*Philine denticulata*	Copepods, *Sagitta* sp.	Pelagic fish including clupeids	Atlantic, western Baltic
Podocotyle atomon	Fish including cod	*Littorina* spp.	Amphipods including *Gammarus* spp. and isopods	NA	Atlantic to southern Baltic
Lepidapedon elongatum	Fish including cod	*Onoba aculeus*	Polychaetes, molluscs	NA	Atlantic, western Baltic
Nematodes					
Anisakis simplex	Cetaceans (whales)	Euphausiaceans, copepods	Clupeids	Cod and other fish species	Atlantic with immigration of infected herring into western Baltic
Pseudoterranova decipiens	Pinnipeds (seals)	Crustaceans (copepods, isopods, amphipods)	Cod	Cod	Atlantic, southern Baltic
Contracaecum osculatum	Pinnipeds (seals)	Copepods, isopods, amphipods	Clupeids and other small fish	Cod	Atlantic to eastern Baltic
Hysterothylacium aduncum	Fish including cod	Crustaceans including copepods	Small fish	Cod, eelpout	Atlantic to eastern Baltic
Capillaria gracilis	Fish including cod	Chironomid larvae, oligochaetes	Sand goby, dab	NA	Atlantic to southern Baltic
Acanthocephalans					
Echinorhynchus gadi	Fish including cod	Amphipods	NA	Various fish species	Atlantic to eastern Baltic
Pomphorhynchus laevis	Fish including cod	Amphipods	NA	?	Atlantic to eastern Baltic
Corynosoma spp.	Pinnipeds (seals)	Amphipods	Fish	Various fish species	Atlantic to eastern Baltic

Table 1.
Parasitic endohelminths with potential as biological indicators.

2. Parasites as indicator species

2.1 Digenean trematodes

The skin fluke *Cryptocotyle lingua* may be applied as an indicator for the western Baltic as this digenean *C. lingua* is a marine organism and infects cod in the western Baltic. The high salinity waters in the western Baltic support survival and reproduction of the common periwinkle *Littorina littorea* which is the first intermediate host of the parasite [15, 22]. It is called the skin fluke of cod and flatfishes, and it elicits black spot disease in these hosts. The life cycle comprises the adult hermaphroditic fluke in the intestine of a fish-eating bird, e.g. a seagull. Eggs from the adult fluke enter the aquatic environment with the host faeces. These eggs are ingested by the marine snail *L. littorea*, which acts as the first intermediate host. In the snail the eggs hatch, and the emerging larvae invade the host snail where new stages, sporocysts and rediae, are produced. Cercariae develop in the rediae, and they are shed into the water where the second intermediate host, e.g. the cod, becomes infected by cercariae. These penetrate the host skin and superficial muscle layers where they attain the metacercarial stage [23]. The host reacts to these parasitic stages by mounting both a cellular and a humoral response. Melanophores gather around the parasite which after some time will be located in the centre of a black spot made of host cells. However, the metacercaria is protected against this immune response by a secreted cyst wall. When the final host, the seagull, eats the infected fish, the fish will be digested, but the parasite will be activated and develop into the adult mature stage in the bird's intestine. This parasite will infect cod in the western part of the Baltic where the intermediate snail host is present but not in the eastern part (because *Littorina littorea* is absent there). Therefore, the parasite can be used as a biological tag [15]. If an infected cod is caught in the eastern Baltic, it can be deduced that it must have been migrating from the infection area in the western Baltic.

The eye flukes within the genus *Diplostomum* comprise various species, and the form occurring in Baltic fishes was originally termed *D. spathaceum* although recent work suggests a more diverse occurrence of species [8]. The eye fluke in the Baltic cod may be used as an indicator for activity in the eastern part of the Baltic. This digenean is a freshwater organism which is commonly found in the eastern part of the Baltic where water is of low salinity [15]. The life cycle includes birds, fish, and molluscs. The first intermediate host is the pulmonate snail, *Lymnaea (Radix) peregra,* which is a freshwater organism. However, it is able to survive in the brackish water in low salinity areas of the northern, eastern, and southern part of the Baltic), but it is absent in the western parts. The second intermediate hosts are fishes, and the final hosts are fish-eating birds. In the bird intestine, the hermaphroditic digenean produces eggs which are shed with host faeces into the aquatic environment. The egg hatches, and the free-living larva, the miracidium, escapes from the egg and locates a host snail. Following penetration of this intermediate host, further development occurs with new larval stages, sporocysts and daughter sporocysts, being produced. In these stages cercariae are produced and are subsequently shed into the water. The furcocercaria penetrates the host skin or gills of the fish host (second intermediate host), sheds the tail, and migrates through the vascular system to the eye lens where the metacercarial stage develops. Following ingestion by a seagull, the fish will be digested, but the flatworm develops into the adult stage in the host intestine. The pyloric trematode *Lepidapedon elongatum* is a marine species infecting the Baltic cod [24]. It obtains maturity in a very specialized part of the gastrointestinal part, the pyloric caeca. Here the hermaphroditic worm produces eggs which are released with the intestinal content to the sea. A mollusc acts as the first intermediate host. Thus, in the marine snail *Onoba aculeus*, the first larval stages (redia) are developed. These release cercariae infective for the second intermediate host, the polychaete *Nereis diversicolor*. Thus, metacercariae encyst in this free-living and bottom-dwelling worm and become infective for the final host, the cod. When the cod feeds on infected polychaetes, it will acquire the infection because the metacercaria excysts and develops to the adult stage in the pyloric caeca of the fish. Thus, infection with this digenean will mirror the marine life and food of the cod. Infected cod caught in more diluted parts of the Baltic (such as the northern Bothnian Bay), where the first intermediate host is lacking, will indicate migration of cod from more saline parts of the Baltic.

Other digeneans such as *Hemiurus lühei* and *Brachyphallus crenatus* can be found in the stomach or intestine of the Baltic cod. They acquire the infection following ingestion of infected clupeids such as sprat and herring [9, 11]. The first intermediate mollusc hosts (*Retusa obtusa* and *Philine denticulata*, respectively) of these two hemiurid trematodes have a western distribution in the Baltic Sea which restrict infection of the second intermediate host (copepods) to the western and southern Baltic Sea [25, 26]. The copepod communities in different parts of the Baltic Sea were mapped by Ackefors [27] showing suitable copepod hosts throughout the area. Feeding on benthic amphipods can be indicated by finding cod infected by the trematode *Podocotyle atomon*. It will further reflect that the cod has been migrating to certain areas with a minimum salinity. Thus, *P. atomon* occurs in the stomach and intestine of Baltic cod if it has been foraging on amphipods (second intermediate host) in an area where the first intermediate host (*L. saxatilis*) is present [28]. This marine snails are found in the western Baltic with a distribution to the island of Bornholm (southern Baltic) but absent in the most eastern areas due to the low salinity there.

2.2 Acanthocephalans

Acanthocephalans comprise a group of endoparasitic worms which are prevalent in the Baltic cod. *Echinorhynchus gadi* is a very common species in the intestine of cod. Heavy infections can be seen in the Baltic cod [29–34], and worm counts of more than 500 worms per fish have been recorded although the mean number per fish often varies from 30 to 60. The intermediate host is amphipods such as various species of *Gammarus*, and the infection level may indicate the extent that the cod feeds on this particular crustacean. Especially flatfishes such as flounder and plaice in the Baltic are found infected with *Pomphorhynchus laevis* [35]. However, other species (cod, trout, eel) can obtain lighter infections with *P. laevis*. The life cycle is rather similar to the one of *E. gadi* applying amphipods as intermediate host. Adult female worms produce eggs which are liberated to the surroundings with host faeces. The oval to fusiform eggs are ingested by an amphipod in which the larva (acanthella stage) is developed. Following ingestion by the fish, the larva reaches the posterior part of the intestine, penetrates the mucosa with its proboscis, attaches in the gut wall, and attains maturity. The intensity in cod is generally very low.

Two species within the genus *Corynosoma* (*C. semerme and C. strumosum*) occur in the Baltic. They can both be found in the body cavity and the intestinal wall of Baltic cod but generally at low intensities. The life cycle includes a seal as final host and an amphipod as first intermediate host [36]. The level of infection will reflect the occurrence of finals hosts (pinnipeds) in the area.

2.3 Nematodes

The so-called herring worm or whale worm *Anisakis simplex* is a marine species which is commonly found in marine waters. It is also found in various fish species in the Baltic but only in certain areas. The life cycle of *A. simplex* is entirely marine and demands stenohaline crustaceans (euphausiids) as intermediate hosts. Whales, fish, copepods, and/or euphausiids are obligate parts of the cycle ([37, 38]). The mature female worms in the stomach of whales produce eggs which are released with whale faeces to the marine waters. In the egg the larva develops and moults twice into the third larval stage which subsequently is liberated [38]. The crustaceans eat the larvae, become infected with larvae in their haemocoel, and will transmit the worm to fish predators. In the fish the larvae will normally coil and take positions in the body cavity, organs, or flesh. If a predatory fish ingests an infected fish, the larvae will be transferred to the former. Following ingestion by the whale (e.g. a porpoise), the larvae moult twice and attain maturity in the final host [38]. The crustacean hosts (euphausiids) demand high salinity and do not live in the Baltic due to the low salinity there. This means that the life cycle of the worm is not performed in the Baltic. Nonetheless cod, herring, pikeperch, and flounder can occasionally be found infected in certain areas of the western and southern parts of the Baltic. This can, however, be readily explained by the seasonal immigration of infected herring from the North Sea into the Baltic. Thus, it is known that a number of herring stocks occur in the Baltic Sea. They are mostly stationary or perform limited migrations within the Baltic. However, one stock, the spring-spawning Rügen herring, is performing long-range migrations. These fish spawn along the coastline of Germany and Poland in the first months of the year. Following this event they swim out of the Baltic to the North Sea where they feed on euphausiids during the summer season. In this period they become infected with numerous anisakids before they migrate through Øresund towards the Baltic in the autumn. During their stay in the Baltic, they are subjected to predation by cod, salmon, pikeperch, and other predatory fish (even flounder). In this way the infection is spread to other species in this brackish sea [37]. In fact, the parasite is not host specific as a larva and is able to infect many fish species.

The cod worm *Pseudoterranova decipiens*, which generally is associated with cod in Atlantic waters [39, 40], has been considered absent from the Baltic cod population for several decades. However, recent parts of the Baltic cod population were found infected [16]. The increasing population of grey seal, which is the final host of the parasite, in the Baltic Sea can explain the increasing occurrence in the western and Baltic parts. The cod worm *P. decipiens* is a marine nematode species within the family Anisakidae. It is commonly found in cod from the Atlantic, but due to the low abundance of suitable final hosts (pinnipeds such as grey seal), it has been absent from the Baltic [41]. In addition, the low salinity in the eastern part of the Baltic does not support the life cycle of the parasite but cod in the western and southern part of the Baltic (around the island Bornholm) where salinity is sufficiently high to support egg hatching and larval survival of the parasite and the infection of cod has increased [16].

The nematode larva *Contracaecum osculatum* invading the liver of Baltic cod is using a seal as the final host [13, 14]. The adult worms copulate in the gastrointestinal tract of the seal. Eggs are passed out with host faeces and embryonate in the sea. Two moults occur in the egg before hatching, and the third-stage larva emerges [42]. This is infective to copepods and smaller crustaceans (transport/paratenic hosts) upon ingestion. Fish predating on these animals become infected with the third-stage larva. Sprat and herring will often act as an important paratenic host as they obtain infection by ingesting third-stage larvae contained in copepods, and cod will then acquire infection when predating on these clupeids [43, 44]. Cod will often carry infections in the liver. When fish are ingested by a marine mammal, such as the seal, the worm will moult twice and attain the adult stage in the stomach of the final host [42]. The highly expanding grey seal population in the Baltic Sea during the latest decades [18, 45] is responsible for a marked increase of infections with *C. osculatum* third-stage larvae in cod livers ([13, 17, 20, 21, 46, 47, 48–50]). It has previously, in the 1950s, during an earlier period with a large Baltic grey seal population, been observed that the liver tissue of Baltic cod became emaciated due to the heavy burdens of *C. osculatum* third-stage larvae [51, 52] exactly as was described during the present epidemic [53]. Occurrence of this nematode larva in Baltic cod is clearly an eminent indicator for occurrence and size of the seal population.

Hysterothyla[cium aduncum is a marine nematode having its adult stage in the fish, e.g. the eelpout, cod, flounder, or sea trout [14, 22, 35], although cod may act as an intermediate/paratenic host as well [54]. Eggs are delivered to the sea, where they infect smaller crustaceans (copepods, amphipods, mysids, isopods) [55] acting as intermediate hosts. Fish become infected by feeding on these intermediate/transport hosts [54]. Smaller fish can obtain infection with third-stage larvae (if the infecting larvae are small at the time of infection) and will transfer the worms to larger predatory fish upon predation. If the larvae at the time of infection are large, the worms will moult twice and attain maturity directly in the fish digestive tract. This parasite is common in the Baltic cod [34, 56] but appears to be less prevalent when compared to the occurrence in North Sea cod [57, 58] and may affect some hosts if they are heavily infected.

The very thin nematode *Capillaria gracilis* has a very wide geographical distribution. Light infections of this species, using the cod as a final host, have been noted in the intestine, mainly rectum, of Baltic cod. Various invertebrates, such as insect larvae of chironomids, are intermediate host [59], and the presence of the parasite in the cod may reflect the ingestion of these invertebrates.

3. Conclusion

The Baltic cod population is vulnerable as it is constantly being exposed to extremely varying hydrographic and biological conditions due to its relatively stationary life cycle in the Baltic Sea. Due to its biological and economical importance of this cod stock, it is monitored and surveyed by the use of classical methodologies within fishery biology. Additional information and higher resolution of parameters, such as local migration within the Baltic and food intake (quantitative and qualitative), will be obtained in a parasitological examination of the fish. It is recommended to include regular parasitological investigation of Baltic cod in future survey programmes. The present work points to use of digenean metacercariae in the cod as indicators of performance in the western Baltic (black spot disease caused by *C. lingua*) and performance in the eastern Baltic (eye fluke disease caused by the genus *Diplostomum*). The presence of intestinal parasites such as the acanthocephalan *E. gadi* reflects the ingestion of amphipods as these crustaceans are obligate intermediate hosts. Occurrence of the anisakid nematode larva *A. simplex* in the flesh, organs, and body cavity of Baltic cod indicates feeding on a specific herring stock. These herrings are migrating seasonally from the North Sea to the Baltic for spawning. The life cycle is not conducted in the Baltic Sea due to the low salinity there, but the import with migrating fish explains the occurrence in stationary Baltic cod. The presence of the cod worm *P. decipiens* and the cod liver worm *C. osculatum* indicates the size of the grey seal population in the Baltic Sea as these nematode species have their adult reproductive stage in the grey seal stomach. The digenean adult hemiurids—comprising *B. crenatus* and *H. luehei*—in the stomach of cod indicate feeding on migrating sprat and herring which have been infected in the western and southern Baltic Sea. The trematode P. atomon occurs in the stomach and intestine of Baltic cod if it has been foraging on amphipods (second intermediate host) in an area where the first intermediate host (*L. saxatilis*) is present. The nematode *Capillaria gracilis* in the rectum of cod indicates that chironomids may be included in the diet of cod. The marine nematode *H. aduncum* (adult in the stomach and intestine) or third-stage larvae in host organs are the least informative species as euryhaline nematode occurs and reproduces in large parts of the Baltic.

Conflict of interest

The author declares that he has no conflict of interest.

Author details

Kurt Buchmann
Laboratory of Aquatic Pathobiology, Faculty of Health and Medical Sciences, University of Copenhagen, Denmark

*Address all correspondence to: kub@sund.ku.dk

References

[1] Herlemann DPR, Labrenz M, Jürgens K, Bertilsson S, Waniek JJ, Andersson AF. Transitions in bacterial communities along the 2000 km salinity gradient of the Baltic Sea. ISME Journal. 2011;5:1571-1579

[2] Bagge O, Thurow F, Steffensen E, Bay J. The Baltic cod. Dana. 1994;**10**:1-28

[3] Hemmingsen W, Mackenzie K. The parasite fauna of the Atlantic cod, *Gadus morhua* L. Advances in Marine Biology. 2001;**40**:1-80

[4] Kabata Z. Parasites as biological tags. International Convention for the Northwest Atlantic Fisheries, Special Publication. 1963;**4**:31-37

[5] MacKenzie K. Parasites as biological tags in population studies of marine organisms: an update. Parasitology. 2002;**124**:153-163. DOI: 10.1017/S0031182002001518

[6] Marcogliese DJ. Food webs and the transmission of parasites to marine fish. Parasitology. 2002;**124**:83-99

[7] Margolis L. Parasites as an auxiliary source of information about the biology of Pacific salmons (genus *Oncorhynchus*). Journal of the Fisheries Research Board of Canada. 1965;**22**:1387-1395

[8] Mehrdana F, Marana MH, Skov J, Bahlool QZM, Sindberg D, Mundeling M, et al. Eye fluke infection status in Baltic cod, *Gadus morhua*, after three decades and their use as ecological indicators. Acta Parasitologica. 2015;**60**(3):423-429

[9] Reimer LW. Digene trematoden und Cestoden der Ostseefische als natürliche Fischmarken. Parasitologische Schriftenreihe. 1970;**20**:1-143

[10] Timi JT. Parasites of Argentine anchovy in the Southwest Atlantic: latitudinal patterns and their use for discrimination of host populations. Journal of Fish Biology. 2003;**63**:90-107

[11] Unger P, Klimpel S, Lang T, Palm HW. Metazoan parasites from herring (*Clupea harengus* L.) as biological indicators in the Baltic Sea. Acta Parasitologica. 2014;**59**:518-528

[12] Williams HH, MacKenzie K, McCarthy AM. Parasites as biological indicators of the population biology, migrations, diet, and phylogenetics of fish. Reviews in Fish Biology and Fisheries. 1992;**2**:144-176

[13] Zuo S, Kania PW, Mehrdana F, Marana MH, Buchmann K. *Contracaecum osculatum* and other anisakid nematodes in grey seals and cod in the Baltic sea: Molecular and ecological links. Journal of Helminthology. 2018;**92**:81-89. DOI: 10.1017/S0022149X17000025

[14] Fagerholm HP. Parasites of Fish in Finland. VI. Nematodes. Acta Academiae Aboensis, B. 1982;**40**:5-128

[15] Buchmann K. Prevalence and intensity of infection of *Cryptocotyle lingua* (Creplin) and *Diplostomum spathaceum* (Rudolphi) – parasitic metacercariae of Baltic cod (*Gadus morhua* L.). Nordisk Veterinaermedicin. 1986b;**38**:303-307

[16] Buchmann K, Kania PW. Emerging *Pseudoterranova decipiens* (Krabbe, 1878) problems in Baltic cod, *Gadus morhua* L., associated with grey seal colonization of spawning grounds. Journal of Fish Diseases. 2012;**35**(11):861-866

[17] Haarder S, Kania PW, Galatius A, Buchmann K. Increased *Contracaecum osculatum* infection in Baltic cod (*Gadus morhua*) livers (1982-2012) associated with increasing grey seal (*Halichoerus*

gryphus) populations. Journal of Wildlife Diseases. 2014;**50**(3):537-543

[18] Lunneryd SG, Bostrom MK, Aspholm PE. Sealworm (*Pseudoterranova decipiens*) infection in grey seals (*Halichoerus grypus*), cod (*Gadus morhua*) and shorthorn sculpin (*Myoxocephalus scorpius*) in the Baltic Sea. Parasitology Research. 2015;**114**:257-264

[19] Mehrdana F, Bahlool QZM, Skov J, Marana MH, Sindberg D, Mundeling M, et al. Occurrence of zoonotic nematodes *Pseudoterranova decipiens*, *Contracaecum osculatum* and *Anisakis simplex* in cod (*Gadus morhua*) from the Baltic Sea. Veterinary Parasitology. 2014b;**205**:581-587

[20] Nadolna K, Podolska M. Anisakid larvae in the liver of cod (*Gadus morhua*) L. from the southern Baltic Sea. Journal of Helminthology. 2014;**88**:237-246

[21] Rodjuk GN. Infestation rates of the main commercial fish species with larva of *Contracaecum osculatum* (Rudolphi, 1802) in Russian waters of the South Baltic in 2000-2012. Parasitologiya. 2014;**48**(3):220-232. (in Russian with English summary)

[22] Möller H, Anders K. Diseases and Parasites of Marine Fishes. Kiel, Germany: Verlag Heino Möller; 1986

[23] Borges JN, Skov J, Bahlool QZM, Møller OS, Kania PW, Santos CP, et al. Viability of *Cryptocotyle lingua* metacercariae from Atlantic cod (*Gadus morhua*) after exposure to freezing and heating in the temperature range from −80-100°C. Food Control. 2015;**50**:371-377

[24] Køie M. On the morphology and life-history of *Lepidapedon elongatum* (Lebour, 1908) Nicoll, 1910 (Trematoda, Lepocreadiidae). Ophelia. 1985;**24**(3):135-153

[25] Køie M. On the morphology and life-history of *Hemiurus Luehei* Odhner, 1905 (Digenea: Hemiuridae). Journal of Helminthology. 1990;**64**:193-202

[26] Køie M. Life cycle and structure of the fish digenean *Brachyphallus crenatus* (Hemiuridae). The Journal of Parasitology. 1992;**78**(2):338-343

[27] Ackefors H. Ecological zooplankton investigations in the Baltic proper 1963-1965. Institute of Marine Research, Lysekil, Fishery Board of Sweden. Series Biology. 1969;**18**:1-138

[28] Køie M. On the morphology and life-history of *Podocotyle reflexa* (Creplin, 1825) Odhner, 1905, and a comparison of its developmental stages with those of *P. atomon* (Rudolphi, 1802) Odhner, 1905 (Trematoda, Opecoelidae). Ophelia. 1981;**20**(1):17-43

[29] Buchmann K. On the infection of Baltic cod (*Gadus morhua* L.) by the acanthocephalan *Echinorhynchus gadi*. Nordisk Veterinaermedicin. 1986a;**38**:308-314

[30] Buchmann K. Variations of the infection level of *Echinorhynchus gadi* (Acanthocephala) in Baltic cod (*Gadus morhua*). Bulletin of the European Association of Fish Pathologists. 1988;**8**:11-14

[31] Buchmann K. Ecological implications of *Echinorhynchus gadi* parasitism of Baltic cod (*Gadus morhua*). Journal of Fish Biology. 1995;**46**:539-540

[32] Nordenberg CB. Ichthyo-parasitological studies on the Baltic cod. Kungliga Fysiografiska Sällskapet i Lund Förhandlingar. 1963;**33**:49-61

[33] Sobecka E, Szostakowska B, MacKenzie K, Hemmingsen W, Prajsnar S, Eydal M. Genetic and morphological variation in Echinorhynchus gadi Zoega in Müller, 1776 (Acanthocephala:

Echinorhynchidae) from Atlantic cod *Gadus morhua* L. Journal of Helminthology. 2012;**86**(1):16-25

[34] Studnicka M. Internal parasites of the cod, *Gadus morhua*L., from Gdansk Bay of the Baltic Sea. Acta Parasitologica Polonica. 1965;**3**:283-290

[35] Thulin J, Höglund J, Lindesjöö E. Fish Diseases in Coastal Waters of Sweden. Stockholm, Sweden: Almänna Förlaget; 1989

[36] Sinisalo T, Valtonen ET. *Corynosoma* acanthocephalans in their paratenic fish hosts in the northern Baltic Sea. Parasite. 2003;**10**(3):227-233

[37] Grabda J. The occurrence of anisakid nematode larvae in Baltic cod (*Gadus morhua callarias* L.) and the dynamics of their invasion. Acta Ichthyologica et Piscatoria. 1976;**6**:3-22

[38] Køie M, Berland B, Burt MDB. Development to third-stage larvae occurs in the eggs of Anisakis simplex and Pseudoterranova decipeins (Nematoda, Ascaridoidea, Anisakidae). Canadian Journal of Fisheries and Aquatic Sciences. 1995;**52**(1):134-139

[39] Brattey J, Bishop CA, Myers RA. Geographic distribution and abundance of *Pseudoterranova decipiens* (Nematoda: Ascaridoidea) in the musculature of Atlantic cod, *Gadus morhua*, from Newfoundland and Labrador. Canadian Bulletin of Fisheries and Aquatic Sciences. 1990;**222**:67-82

[40] McClelland G. The trouble with sealworms (*Pseudoterranova decipiens* species complex, Nematoda): A review. Parasitology. 2002;**124**:S183-S203

[41] Myjak P, Szostakowska B, Wojciechowski J, Pietkiewicz H, Rokicki J. Anisakid larvae in cod from the southern Baltic Sea. Archive of Fishery and Marine Research. 1994;**42**:149-161

[42] Køie M, Fagerholm HP. The life-cycle of *Contracaecum osculatum* (Rudolphi, 1802) *sensu stricto* (Nematoda, Ascaridoidea, Anisakidae) in view of experimental infections. Parasitology Research. 1995;**81**:481-489

[43] Skrzypczak M, Rolbiecki L. Endoparasitic Helminths of the European Sprat, *Sprattus sprattus* (Linnaeus, 1758) from the gulf of Gdansk (the Southern Baltic Sea) with a checklist of its parasites. Russian Journal of Marine Biology. 2015;**41**:167-175

[44] Zuo S, Huwer B, Bahlool Q, Al-Jubury A, Daugbjerg Christensen N, Korbut R, et al. Host size-dependent anisakid infection in Baltic cod *Gadus morhua* associated with differential food preferences. Diseases of Aquatic Organisms. 2016;**120**:69-75

[45] Skrzypczak M, Rokicki J, Pawliczka I, Najda K, Dzido J. Anisakids of seals found on the southern coast of Baltic Sea. Acta Parasitologica. 2014;**59**:165-172

[46] Mehrdana F, Bahlool QZM, Skovgaard A, Kuhn JA, Kania PW, Munk P, Buchmann K. Annual and spatial variability in endo- and ectoparasite infections of North Sea cod (Gadus morhua Linnaeus, 1758) larvae, post-larvae and juveniles. Acta Parasitologica. 2014;**59**(2):284-293

[47] Perdiguero-Alonso D, Montero F, Raga JA, Kostadinova A. Composition and structure of the parasite faunas of cod, *Gadus morhua* L. (Teleostei: Gadidae) in the North East Atlantic. Parasites & Vectors. 2008;**1**(1):-18

[48] Eero M, Hjelm J, Behrens J, Buchmann K, Cardinale M, Casini M, et al. Eastern Baltic cod in distress: biological changes and challenges for stock assessment. ICES Journal of Marine Science. 2015;**72**(8):2180-2186

[49] Horbowy J, Podolska M, Nadolna-Ałtyn K. Increasing occurrence of anisakid nematodes in the liver of cod (*Gadus morhua*) from the Baltic Sea: does infection affect the condition and mortality of fish? Fisheries Research. 2016;**179**:98-103

[50] Sokolova M, Buchmann K, Huwer B, Kania PW, Krumme U, Galatius A, et al. Spatial patterns in infection of cod *Gadus morhua* with the seal-associated liver worm *Contracaecum osculatum* from the Skagerrak to the central Baltic Sea. Marine Ecology Progress Series. 2018;**606**:105-118

[51] Getsevitjute S. Seasonal parasitic infection of Baltic cod liver. Trudy Akademii Nauk Litouskoj SSR Series B. 1955;**2**(1955):127-129. In Russian

[52] Petrushevski GK, Shulman GG. Infection of Baltic cod liver with roundworms. Trudy Akademii Nauk Litouskoj SSR Series B. 1955;**2**(1955): 119-125. (in Russian)

[53] Buchmann K, Mehrdana F. Effects of anisakid nematodes *Anisakis simplex* (s.l.), *Pseudoterranova decipiens* (s.l.) and *Contracaecum osculatum* (s.l.) on fish and consumer health. Food and Waterborne Parasitology. 2016;**4**:13-22

[54] Køie M. Aspects of the life cycle and morphology of *Hysterothylacium aduncum* (Rudolphi, 1802) (Nematoda, Ascaridoidea, Anisakidae). Canadian Journal of Zoology. 1993;**71**(7):1289-1296

[55] Pawlak J, Nadolna-Ałtyn K, Szostakowska B, Pachur M, Podolska M. *Saduria entomon* infected with *Hysterothylacium aduncum* found in situ in the stomach of cod (*Gadus morhua*) from the Baltic Sea. Journal of Helminthology. 2018;**92**:645-648

[56] Pilecka-Rapacz M, Sobecka E. Parasites of young Baltic cod, *Gadus morhua callarias* L. in the Gulf of Puck, Poland. Acta Ichthyologica et Piscatoria. 2004;**34**(2):235-240

[57] Mehrdana F, Bahlool QZM, Skovgaard A, Kuhn JA, Kania PW, Munk P, et al. Annual and spatial variability in endo- and ectoparasite infections of North Sea cod (*Gadus morhua* Linnaeus, 1758) larvae, post-larvae and juveniles. Acta Parasitologica. 2014a;**59**(2):284-293

[58] Skovgaard A, Bahlool QZM, Munk P, Berge T, Buchmann K. Infection of North Sea cod, *Gadus morhua* L., larvae with the parasitic nematode *Hysterothylacium aduncum* Rudolphi. Journal of Plankton Research. 2011;**33**:1311-1316

[59] Køie M. The life-cycle of *Capillaria gracilis* (Capillariidae), a nematode parasite of gadoid fish. Marine Biology Research. 2001;**86**:383-387